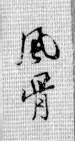

风骨

图书在版编目（CIP）数据

风骨 : 汉英对照 / 李铁军编著 ; 黄慧萍译 .
-- 北京 : 五洲传播出版社 , 2023.10
ISBN 978-7-5085-5121-0

Ⅰ . ①风… Ⅱ . ①李… ②黄… Ⅲ . ①显微摄影－医学摄影－摄影集
Ⅳ . ① R445-64

中国国家版本馆 CIP 数据核字 (2023) 第 192537 号

风骨

显微摄影： 李铁军
编著 / 翻译： 李铁军　黄慧萍
英文审定： 刘式南
出 版 人： 关　宏
责任编辑： 苏　谦
助理编辑： 阴溁萌
装帧设计： 北京正视文化艺术有限责任公司
出版发行： 五洲传播出版社
地　　址： 北京市海淀区北三环中路 31 号生产力大楼 B 座 6 层
邮　　编： 100088
发行电话： 010-82005927，010-82007837
网　　址： www.cicc.org.cn，www.thatsbooks.com
印　　刷： 河北京平诚乾印刷有限公司
版　　次： 2023 年 10 月第 1 版第 1 次印刷
开　　本： 889mm×1194mm　1/20
印　　张： 13
定　　价： 139.00 元

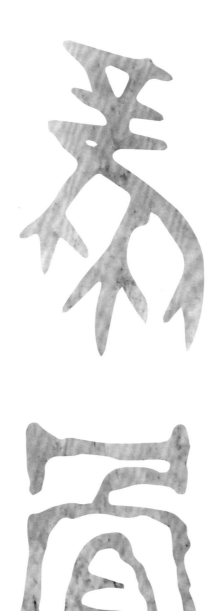

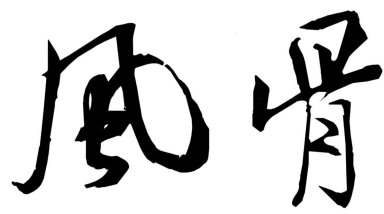

风骨
Backbone

显微摄影：李铁军

编著：李铁军 黄慧萍

Photomicrographed by Li Tiejun

Written and edited by Li Tiejun and Huang Huiping

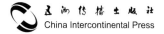

五洲传播出版社
China Intercontinental Press

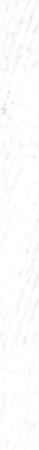

Backbone

骨

Backbone

序

风骨百年，心笔行书

李铁军

北京大学口腔医学院 教授

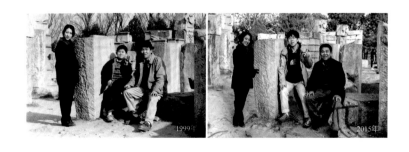

骨是人和脊椎动物体内支持身体、保护内脏的坚硬组织器官。人有206块骨，虽然很多是左右对称骨，但每一块骨头都不一样。

人从生到死，骨的变化一刻都没有停止过。人从小变大，由矮变高，长大成人，经历岁月沧桑，骨则从密变疏，由直变曲……我们容易看到的是容颜、体貌的改变，却常常不觉藏于皮肉深处的骨的变化。

骨之于生命，可谓默默撑持、忍辱负重、生死相随。然而，中国人对骨却有截然不同的诠释和隐喻。

首先，来看广为人们接受的世俗生死观。至今仍有很多人相信，没有皮肉的骨头（骷髅）是鬼，有骨有肉方为人。人们对肉身的眷恋，从各类帝王贵族古墓保护尸体的宝典秘籍中便可略见一斑，如棺木材料、密封技术、液体沁涂、金缕玉身，等等，为的就是骨肉不离，虽死犹生。著名的《鬼趣图》题诗中便有"对面不知人有骨，到头方信鬼无皮"的名句，可见，肉与骨的区分，成了生与死、人与鬼的隐喻。家喻户晓的《西游记》中的角色白骨精，更是把骨与邪、毒、魔、妖勾连到极致。巧扮妖媚的女妖迷惑唐僧，花言巧语，令其险些丧命，最后被神通广大的孙悟空棒打三回才终现原形。"白骨"是何等的恐怖！这也难怪，就连我这样学医出身的人，面对解剖室内的骷髅标本时，内心也有一丝难以躲闪的寒意。

不过，中国人对骨的敬畏和赞扬也是无处不在的。比如"铁骨""傲骨""仙骨""风骨"等词语，常把人带入一种超凡脱俗的雅境。这类文字表达好像在汉语中尤为特别、独树一帜。在我试图把这些有关骨的词语翻译成英文时，着实很难找到贴切的表达词汇。这里很可能有其深刻的历史文化意涵，也反映了中国人对自然和生命的独特感悟。

我不禁想到"甲骨文"——这种我们可辨识的最早的成熟汉字。据古文字专家考证，这些商朝晚期刻于龟甲或兽骨之上的"殷墟文字"，已具备了中国书法的用笔、结字、章法三要素。这说明作为一种象形文字，汉字很早便不只是一种简单的记录工具，它同时也是艺术。而在其他文明中，文字的字母化则是走上了另一条不同的路径。这些古汉字刻在骨上，便有了个性、气质、神韵和活力，于是在后来汉语的艺术语境中，常遇到与骨相关联的词汇便不奇怪了。

在中国书法史上留下光辉篇章的魏晋书法、唐宋书法，更是将"骨"作为其审美的重要考量。在魏晋南北朝时期，人们将"骨""气""力"结合在一起，形成所谓"风骨"，并以此来评判一个人，这表明这个时代已注重对个人独立精神和行为举止的品鉴，而不是局限于人的五官外貌。后来"风骨"这一概念不断延伸，除了用于描写人的品格和气质，也指书法、绘画和文学作品的风格有个性、有力量。例如唐代书法家中，颜真卿的字浑厚饱满，柳公权的字清秀苍劲，两人堪称楷书的顶峰和典范，在书法史上被称之为"颜筋柳骨"，传承千年。这种具有时代特征的美学思想，把"风骨"一词引入书法的审美追求，其中"骨力"反映的是书法内在的力量，并非一定要剑拔弩张，而是由内而外，既有力，又秀气，挺拔而有风格。

骨之所以还引申指人的品质、气概等，除了因为它在"生"时对生命的支撑和保护，还在于它在"死"后对生命的那份执着和坚守。人生不过百年，我们的肉身终将随生命的终结而回归自然，当那些曾经的"小鲜肉""心肝宝贝"很快丢盔卸甲、随风而去之后，即使又过了很久很久，当年很少抛头露面的"硬骨头"仍在顽强地抵御着自然界的侵蚀，默默讲述着有关生命岁月兴衰和变迁的故事。据说如埋在土里，人骨可存留上千年。所以，考古学家才能通过收集、分析这些人类遗骨，推演出当时人类的生活状态和族群变迁。骨的这种死而不屈、执意为绚丽人生雕刻时光留痕的品质，浸透眷恋、温情，令人敬畏、感慨。希望长生不老，渴望永世不朽，一直是人类的痴念，现在看人体中唯一能与这份痴念稍稍接近一点的便是这把"白骨"。虽然现在的丧葬习俗已变，但即使成灰，骨之于人所蕴含的那种精神气质是不变的。

如果说岩石是地球的"化石"，骨便可以当之无愧地被誉为人的"化石"。

然而，由于在生活状态下骨的"深藏不露"，一般能观察到的"骨的气象"是十分有限的。因工作关系，我常要使用显微镜来观察人的器官、组织和细胞，其中包括骨组织。透过显微镜，将其放大数十倍或数百倍后，骨的万般风姿便赫然显现。它时而坚硬似铁，时而轻柔如风，时而热烈似火，时而宁静如水，有的绚烂而张扬，有的悠远而神秘，仿佛演绎了身体和生命的这场迷局，从无到有、由简至繁、伟岸而立、风雨沧桑、繁华随风、逝水流年、从拥有变成失去，生命里一刻未停止过变化的骨组织，所留下的痕迹是最多的，也是最久远的。

有人说：树没有前途，才在躯干上留下年轮。或许，被华丽皮囊包裹其中的骨也正是如此吧。显微镜下所呈现出的浓淡深浅、光色交融的骨骼微像，像是帮助我们完成了一次富于哲理的视觉抵达，它们与前面提到的"风骨"一词的寓意竟如此地不谋而合，不能不让我们感叹天地造化与道法自然的主客观统一，体悟中华文化的博大精深。这些透过科学棱镜窥探到的骨骼微像，非常生动地诠释了生命的奇迹，以变化万千的难忘瞬间，倾诉这段生命旅程中的所有苦难与幸福。

至此，要回到《风骨》这本书的创作初衷了。当我的显微影像库中这些表现骨的影像越积越多时，我想以"风骨"为题出本画册。然而，单纯的显微影像图册似乎不足以表达"风骨"二字的丰富内涵，于是我便与夫人黄慧萍一起策划了一种全新的呈现方式。我们由"骨"联想到"字"，由生命联想到百年，何不邀请一百个人，从不满周岁的婴儿到百岁老翁，一岁一人，每人书写一词或一句（有时也有两人同写相同词句的情况），文字与骨的显微影像呼应呈现，使这本画册变成由上百人参与的集体创作？除了年龄上的考虑，对这一百多位朋友的选择并无特殊，他们就是芸芸众生中的普通人。当然，这些手稿的募集，离不开身边亲人朋友们的支持、帮助。这样，便有了不会拿笔婴儿的脚印、刚会拿笔幼童的乱划、刚会写字小朋友的稚笔、青少年学生的工整笔迹、大学生和研究生们的激扬文字、中壮年朋友们的信手拈来、老年朋友们的老骥伏枥，还有百岁老人的悠然所乐……

于是，整理百幅骨骼显微影像作品和收集百人行书手稿的这段创作过程，演变成一场非常特别的"行为艺术"。

当我们把这些彼此并无特殊关联的笔迹与富于表现力的一百幅显微图像放在一起时，我们自己也惊呆了。这个百人集体所表现出的精神力量，沿岁月长河奔腾流淌，它们与这些风姿百态的骨骼微像交相辉映，构成"天地人"奇妙的生命交响！除了根据这百幅影像选择了一百个对应的汉语词句外，编者并没有刻意邀请书法家，也没有对书写者做字体或款式的限定，可谓字无定式、随心而书，意在突显"一百个哈姆雷特"式的个性表达。清代文学家刘熙载在《艺概·书概》中曾这样描述："书，如也，如其学，如其才，如其志，总之曰如其人而已。"尽管这里我们收集的并不是书法作品，但"字"如其人，百幅行书便是百人天趣，纵跨百岁就是生命划痕。这些不能称为"书法"的普通字迹符号，仿佛突然获得了感人的呼唤能量，一遍一遍地试图唤醒已沉寂在这些骨骼微像里的生命无声之音、无形之相。这，不正是我一直执着于有关生命的显微摄影创作的初衷吗？

在生命和时间面前，人变得平等和真诚。

意大利作家伊塔洛·卡尔维诺在小说《看不见的城市》中曾这样写道：人活百年，草木数百年，石头千年，但最终只有记忆能帮助我们穿越生死，跨越地狱天堂。我想，人在一生中不断地书写，骨骼在一生中不停地重塑，正是为加深这种"记忆"而展现的本能吧。

这里，我要衷心感谢我的合编者黄慧萍，她是这场"行为艺术"的操盘手，不仅支持鼓励我，还共同策划、具体实施，默默体味其中甘苦。感谢我们的亲人朋友和他们的亲人朋友，特别是我的同学周桂兰教授、我的学生董青主任等。我们一起，才构筑起这个难以组成的百人方阵，尽管其中多数人互不相识，却因我痴心捕捉的显微骨像汇集到一起，以个人的心笔行书，共同编写这本感悟生命和时间的百年风骨画集。感谢你们为这场"风骨"的生命交响所演奏的每个音符。

人生如逆旅，我们都是过客。一如那首相传为仓央嘉措所作的诗：那一世，我转山转水转佛塔，不为修来世，只为在途中与你相见。

天地光阴，匆匆百年。从那一刻，那一天，那一年开始，我们为这本书结缘相聚。假如你相信因果，就让我们祝愿有缘人终将一世相伴和厮守。

2023 年 6 月

Preface
Centenarian backbone and soul-inspired handwriting

Li Tiejun

Professor, Peking University School of Stomatology

Bones are hard tissues and organs supporting the body and protect internal organs in humans and other vertebrates. A person has 206 bones. Although many of them are symmetrical, each bone is different.

From birth to death, bones never stop changing and remodeling. People grow up from small to large, from short to tall. After years of vicissitudes, human bones change from dense to sparse, from straight to curved... What we can easily see is the change of face and body appearance, but we often fail to perceive the change of bones beneath the skin in the depths of flesh.

To life, bones can be described as silently supporting our body, enduring hardships and bearing heavy burdens until death. However, Chinese people have different interpretations and metaphors about bones.

First, let's look at the widely accepted secular view of life and death. So far, many people still believe that bones (or skeletons) without skin and flesh are ghosts, and that a body can be human only when it has both bones and flesh. People's obsession with the fleshy body was reflected in the techniques adopted to protect corpses in ancient emperors' and aristocrats' tombs, such as coffin materials, sealing technology, liquid smear, golden/jade clothing, and so on, which help keep the flesh and bones together, so that they would still look alive. There is a famous line in the poem inscribed in the painting "Ghost's Fun": "You could hardly see the bone behind the face; eventually, you will realize a ghost has no skin". Therefore, the distinction between flesh and bone has become a metaphor for life and death, humans and ghosts. White Bone Demon, a well-known character in the famous

Chinese novel *Journey to the West*, best illustrates the association between bones and the wicked, ruthless devil and demon. She skillfully disguised herself as a poor country girl to confuse the Tang Monk and talked sweet words, which cheated and nearly killed him. Finally, she was beaten three times by the Monkey King before finally showing her original shape of white skeleton. What a terror! It's no wonder that even a medical doctor like me has an involuntary chilling fear when facing the skeleton specimens in the anatomy room.

However, Chinese people's respect and praise for bones are omnipresent. For example, words such as "iron bone", "unyielding bone", "immortal bone" and "backbone" often evoke an extraordinarily artistic and elegant feeling. This kind of expression seems to be particularly characteristic and unique of Chinese. When I tried to translate these "bone" words into English, it proved really difficult to find appropriate equivalents to them. It is very likely that these words have profound historical and cultural implications, and reflect Chinese people's unique perception of nature and life.

It also prompts me to think of "oracle bone inscriptions," the earliest mature Chinese characters we can recognize. According to experts specializing in textual research of ancient characters, these "Yin Ruins characters" carved on tortoise shells or animal bones in the late Shang Dynasty (1600-1046 BC) already had the three essential elements of Chinese calligraphy — strokes, structure and textual composition. This indicates that as a kind of hieroglyphics, Chinese characters were not only a simple recording tool, but also an art at the same time. In other cultures, however, their scripts embarked on a different path through alphabetization. When these ancient Chinese characters were engraved on bones, they began to possess personality, temperament, charm and vitality. Therefore, it is not unusual that one sees so many words related to bones in the Chinese artistic context.

The calligraphy of Wei (220-265) and Jin (265-420) Dynasties, which left a glorious chapter in the history of Chinese calligraphy, takes "bone" as its important aesthetic consideration. In the Wei, Jin and Northern and Southern Dynasties (420-589), people thought that bone, spirit and strength combined to form a man's "feng", or demeanor, which was used to evaluate his integrity and temperament. It shows that during that period, people had already paid attention to the evaluation of a person's independent spirit and behavior, rather than people's superficial looks only. Later, this concept continued extending. Generally, it is used to describe people's tenacious character and temperament, and also to denote that a calligraphy, painting, or literary work has personality and strength. For instance, in Tang Dynasty (618-907), Yan Zhenqing's calligraphy was thick and full, while Liu Gongquan's calligraphy was elegant and vigorous. They are regarded as the peak and model of regular script in Chinese calligraphy. The styles of Yan and Liu were compared to "tendon" and "bone" respectively in the history of calligraphy and have been passed on for thousands of years. This aesthetic thought with the characteristics of the times and culture introduced the word "backbone" into the aesthetic pursuit of calligraphy. Among the terms, "the power of bone" reflects the internal strength of calligraphy. It does not have to be bellicose and menacing, but from the inside to the outside, it is powerful, delicate, and vigorous with style.

The reason why bones have been chosen to represent people's quality and spirit lies in its unyielding hold of life after a human is dead, in addition to its role of sustaining and protecting life when the man is alive. The human life span is roughly a hundred years, and our flesh will dissolve and return to the nature with the ending of life. When the once beautiful "fresh face" and "sweetheart" easily succumb to the Reaper's Scythe and vanish in the wind, the "hard bones," which rarely appear in public in man's living years, still tenaciously resist the erosion of nature and silently adhere to the story of the rise and fall of life. It is said that if buried in earth, human bones can last for thousands of years. That makes it possible for archaeologists to collect and analyze these human remains to deduce the living conditions and ethnic changes of human beings at that time. This spirit of bones refusing to succumb to death and sticking to the trace of the once gorgeous life is awe-inspiring. Pursuing immortality has always been an obsessive desire of human beings. Now, the only thing in the human body that can be somewhat close to this obsession is the "white bones". Although the funeral custom has changed nowadays, even if the body is burned to ashes, the spiritual temperament contained in bones remains unchanged.

If rocks are the "fossil" of the Earth, then the bones well deserve to be called the "fossil" of human.

However, due to the "concealment" of bones in normal conditions, it is rare to see the "image of bones". Because of my medical profession, I often use a microscope to observe human organs, tissues, and cells, including bone tissues. Under the microscope, which magnifies the object dozens or hundreds of times, bone tissues appear impressively in various forms. They look sometimes as hard as iron, and sometimes as gentle as wind; sometimes as vehement as fire, and sometimes as serene as water; sometimes glamorous and flaunting, and sometimes distant and mysterious as if they are trying to relate the whole mysterious story of the body and life, from void to substance, from simplicity to complexity, standing strong, experiencing ups and downs, withering with the passing years, and vanishing into the air. The bone tissues that have never stopped changing for a single while in life have also left the most and longest tracing marks of itself.

Some people say that trees have no way ahead, so they leave ring marks in their trunks. Perhaps the same is true of the bones wrapped in skin and flesh. The microscopic images of bones with rich and variable light and colors seem to be shedding light on our philosophical journey to the visual destination. They coincide with the metaphorical meaning of "backbone" so closely that we can't help marveling at the charm of Taoism in its unity of subjective and objective worlds, and appreciating the profound thinking of Chinese culture. These photomicrographs of bones seen through the prism of science vividly interpret the miracles of life. The captured images of the bones appear to tell the stories about all the suffering and happiness in the human lifetime.

Now, I would like to get back to my original intention of writing this book. When there were more and more images showing the beauty of bones in my files, I developed an idea to publish a special album of these bone images. However, a simple photomicrograph album does not seem enough to convey the rich connotation of the word "backbone". So together with my wife Huang Huiping, I planned a brand-new way of presenting the micro beauty of bones. We thought about the association between "bone" and "handwriting", and between "a living life" and "a hundred years". Why not invite 100 people, from a newborn infant to a centenarian, and invite each of them to write a word or a sentence (occasionally two people write the same words or sentences) which echoes the photomicrographs of bones? This can turn the album into a collective creation participated by more than a hundred people. Except for age consideration, selection of the participants was random.

They are ordinary people among the meat and potatoes crowd from all walks of life. Undoubtedly, the collection of these handwritings would not have been possible without the support and help from our relatives and friends. In this way, we got the footprints of babies who could not hold a pen, the scribbles of toddlers who had just had a try on the pen, the childish works of children who had just learned to write, the neat handwriting of teenagers, the youthful and energetic texts of college / graduate students, the handy writing of middle aged friends, the sophisticated calligraphy of the aged friends, and the leisurely and free scripts of centenarians…

Therefore, the process of sorting hundreds of photomicrographic bone images and collecting hundreds of handwritings became a very special "performance art".

We were stunned when we put these mutually unrelated handwriting works side-by-side with the 100 impressive microscopic images. The spiritual power emanating from this group of 100 people flows like rushing torrents in the river of times. The scripts and the bone images added radiance to each other, forming a wonderful scene of harmonious co-existence of "heaven, earth and human"! We selected 100 Chinese words or sentences which we thought closely match the 100 micrographic images. But we did not intentionally invite professional calligraphers, nor was there any restriction on the font or style of the handwritings by these participants. It can be said that any handwriting was amorphous and followed the writer's own will, which is intended to highlight the possible personal expression of "one hundred Hamlets". Liu Xizai, a writer in Qing Dynasty (1616-1911) once described, this in his book: "handwriting (calligraphy) is like a mirror, which reflects one's knowledge, talent, ambition, and in general one's own self." Although the handwritings we collected here may not be calligraphy works, each of the scripts faithfully mirrors the person who wrote it. All the 100 scripts represent the natural emotions of the 100 people, and the age span of 100 years is the tracing marks of life. These ordinary pictographic characters, which may not be called "calligraphy", seem to have suddenly obtained a touching energy, trying to awaken the silent and invisible life that has been quietly hidden in these micro bone images. Isn't that exactly my original intention that drove me to persistently take micrographic photos to present the beauty of life?

In front of life and time, people become equal and sincere.

Italian writer Italo Calvino once wrote in his novel *Invisible Cities* that people may live for a hundred years, plants or trees for hundreds of years, and stones for thousands of years, but ultimately only memory can help us to go through life and death and to transcend the hell and heaven. I think it must be out of instinct that people keep writing and bones keep reshaping themselves throughout the whole life in order to cement this kind of "memory".

Here, I would like to sincerely thank my co-author, Huang Huiping, who acted as the supervisor of this "performance art". She not only supported and encouraged me in the project, but also joined me for its planning and implementation, for all the joys and hardships involved in it. My thanks go to our relatives and friends and their relatives and friends, especially my classmate Prof. Zhou Guilan and my student Dr. Dongqing. Together, we composed this 100-people formation that is difficult to form. Although most of them did not know each other, the photomicrographs of bones that I captured seem to bring them together to complete this collection of a hundred handwritings matching a hundred images of bones. This album then becomes a life symphony of "Backbone" that truly embodies life and time. Our gratitude goes to every contributor in this collection.

Life is like a journey through all adversities in which we are all passers-by. As the famous poem reportedly written by Tsangyang Gyatso says: Once for a lifetime, I journeyed around mountains, rivers and stupas, not to seek rebirth, but to meet you on the way.

A hundred years is a hasty split second in the context of heaven and earth. From that moment, that day, that year, we have the luck to get together for composition of this book. If you believe in cause and effect, let's wish all travelers in the long journey of life find the companionship and togetherness of predestined partners.

July, 2023

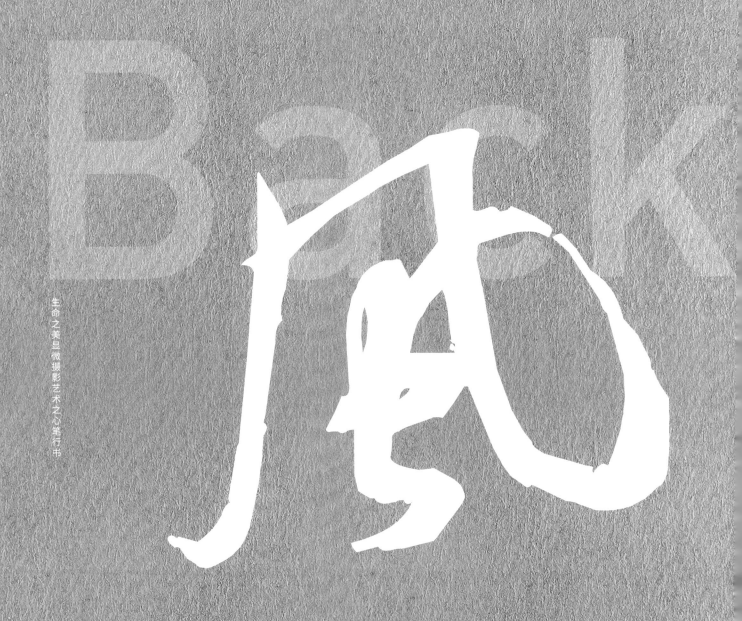

生命之美显微摄影艺术之心笔行书

宵

远古 No.1

未脱钙骨及纤维组织磨片，X40，明视野 + 偏振光，2020

Remote ancient times No.1

Bone and fibrous tissues, Ground section, X40, Light field
+ polarized light, 2020

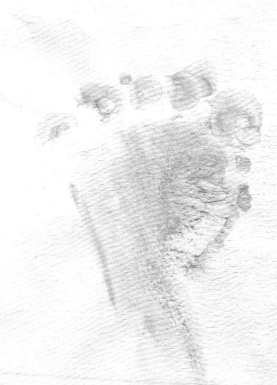

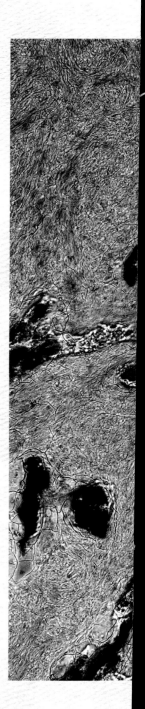

脚印

吴羽希，0 岁

Foot print

Wu Yuxi, 1 Month old

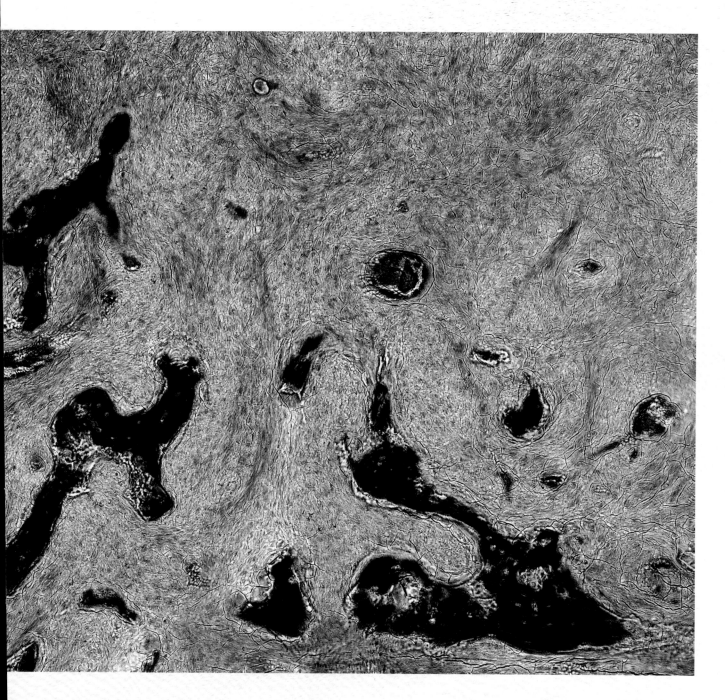

植体的梦想 No.13

未脱钙骨组织和种植体磨片，X100，明视野，2019

Dream of implant No.13

Trabecular bone and implanta, Ground section, X100, Light field, 2019

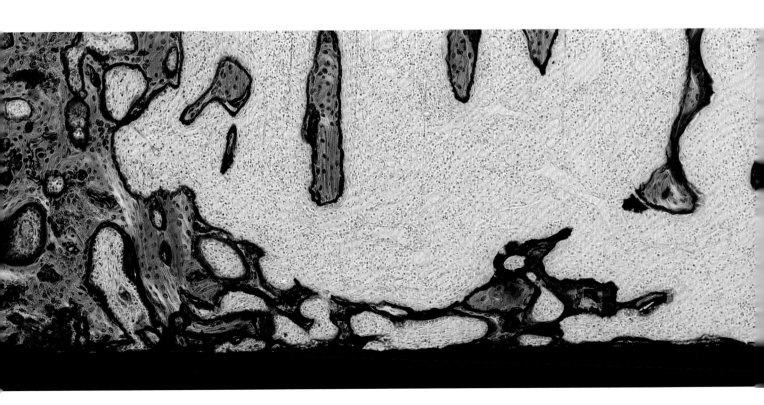

乱划

王若霖，1岁
洪子清，2岁

Drawing

Wang Ruolin, 1 year old
Hong Ziqing, 2 years old

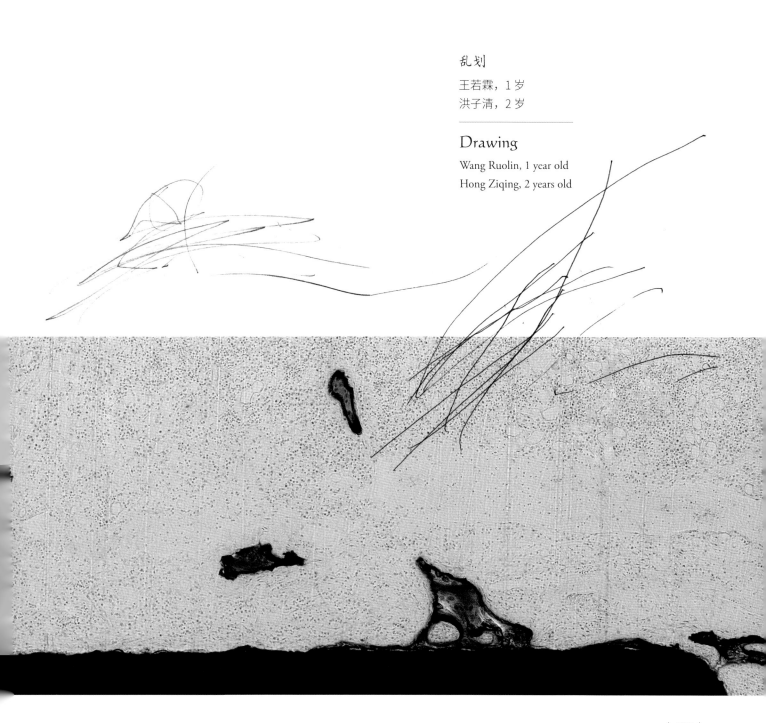

鸟语

脱钙骨组织切片，X100，明视野，2012

Singing bird

Trabecular bone, Tissue section, X100, Light field, 2012

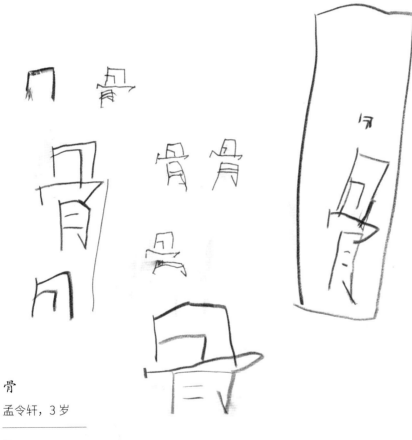

骨

孟令轩，3 岁

Bone

Meng Lingxuan, 3

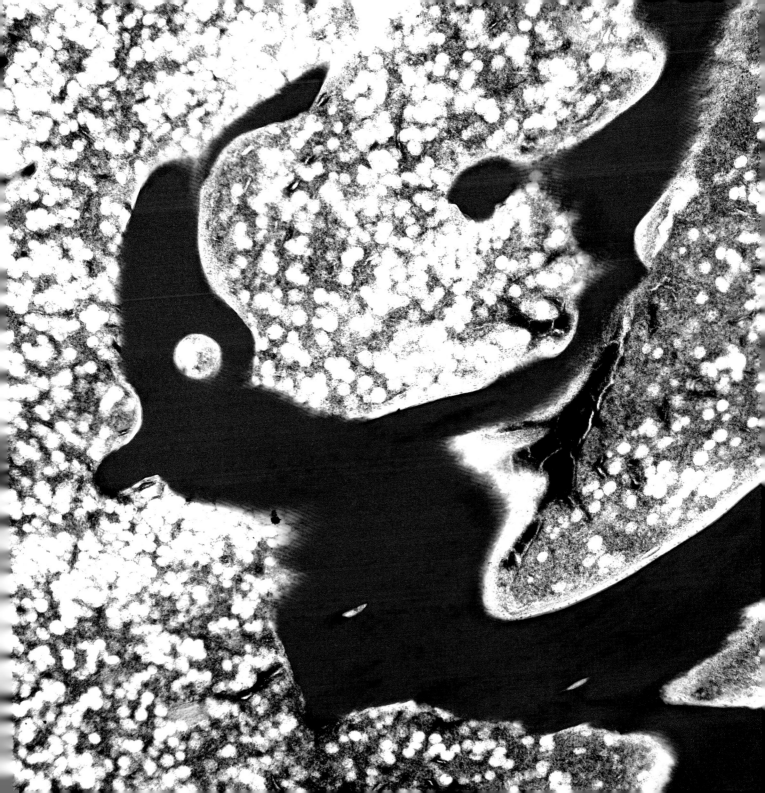

星球 No.5

未脱钙骨组织磨片，X40，明视野 + 偏振光，2020

Planet No.5

Trabecular bone, Ground section, X40, Light field + polarized light, 2020

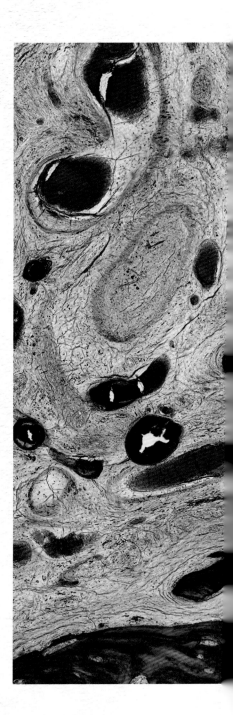

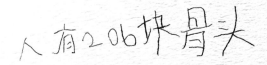

人有 206 块骨头

土千羽，4 岁

There are 206 pieces of bone in a person.

Wang Qianyu, 4

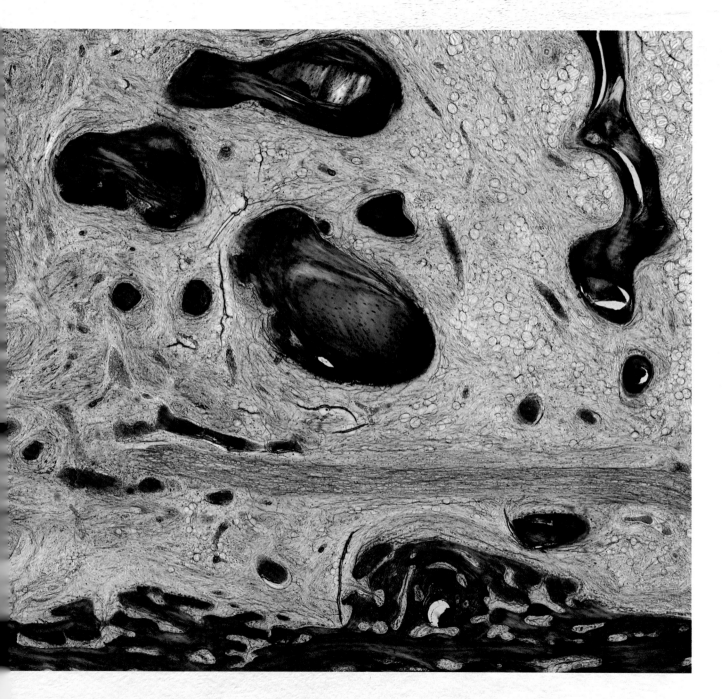

天书 No.164

未脱钙骨组织磨片，X40，明视野 + 偏振光，2020

Heavenly script No.164

Trabecular bone, Ground section, X40, Light field + polarized light, 2020

长高

侯铭禹，5 岁

Growing tall

Hou Mingyu, 5

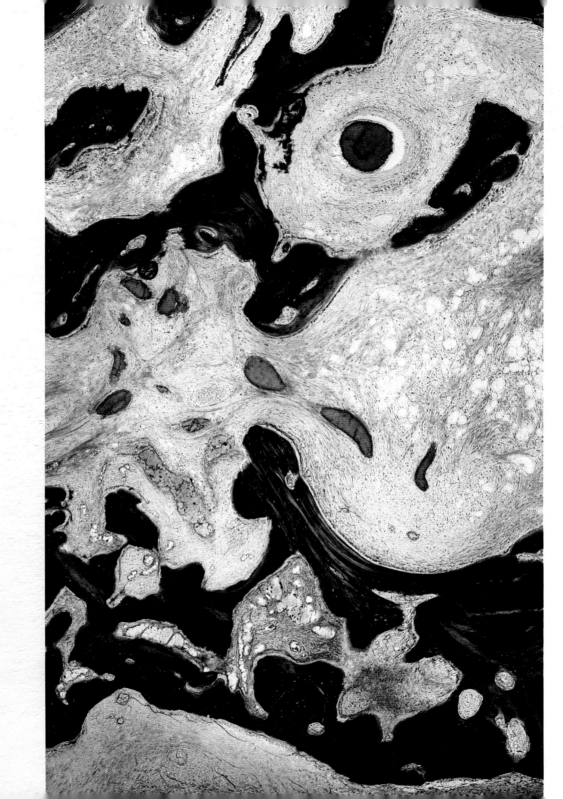

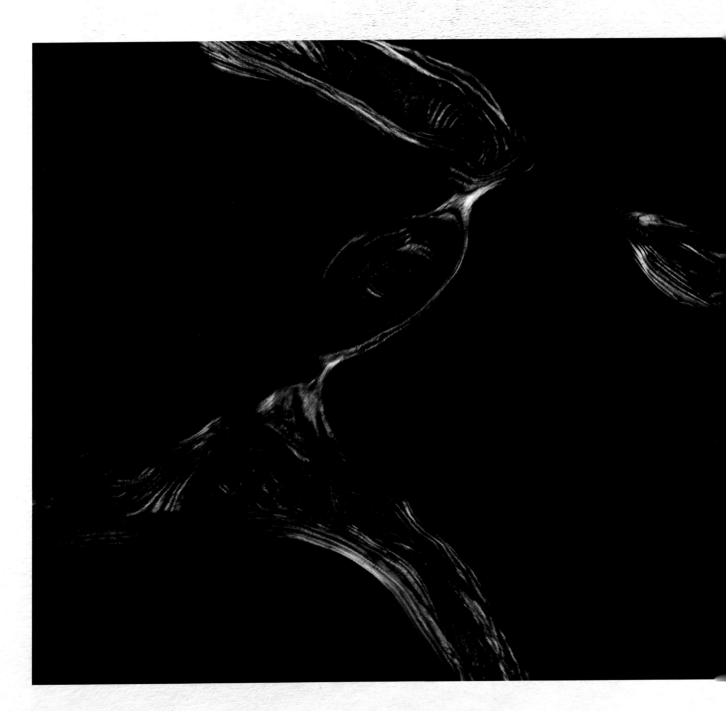

奔

脱钙骨组织切片，X100，偏振光，2014

Running

Trabecular bone, Tissue section, X100, Polarized light, 2014

奔跑

奔跑

曹可毅，6 岁

杨泰，6 岁

Running

Cao Keyi, 6

Yang Tai, 6

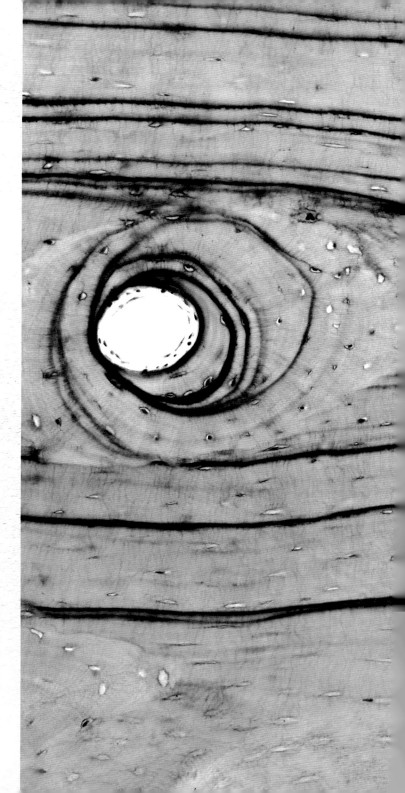

痕迹

脱钙骨组织切片，X200，明视野，2011

Traces

Trabecular bone, Tissue section, X200, Light field, 2011

大眼睛

大眼睛

董博文，7 岁

———

Big eyes

Dong Bowen, 7

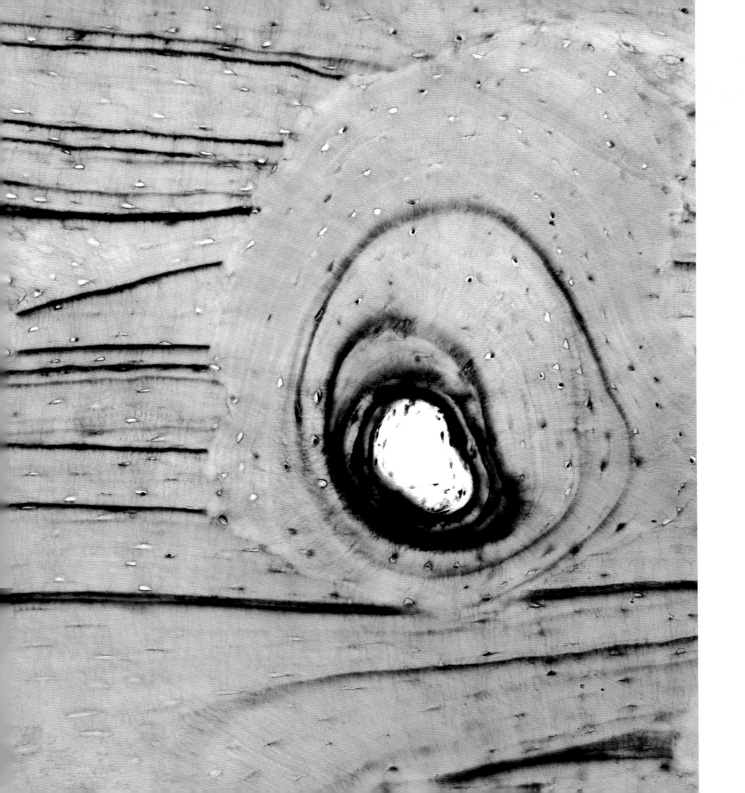

天书 No.114

未脱钙骨组织磨片，X200，明视野 + 偏振光，2019

Heavenly script No.114

Trabecular bone, Ground section, X200, Light field + polarized light, 2019

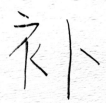

补钙

王若曦，8 岁

Calcium supplement

Wang Ruoxi, 8

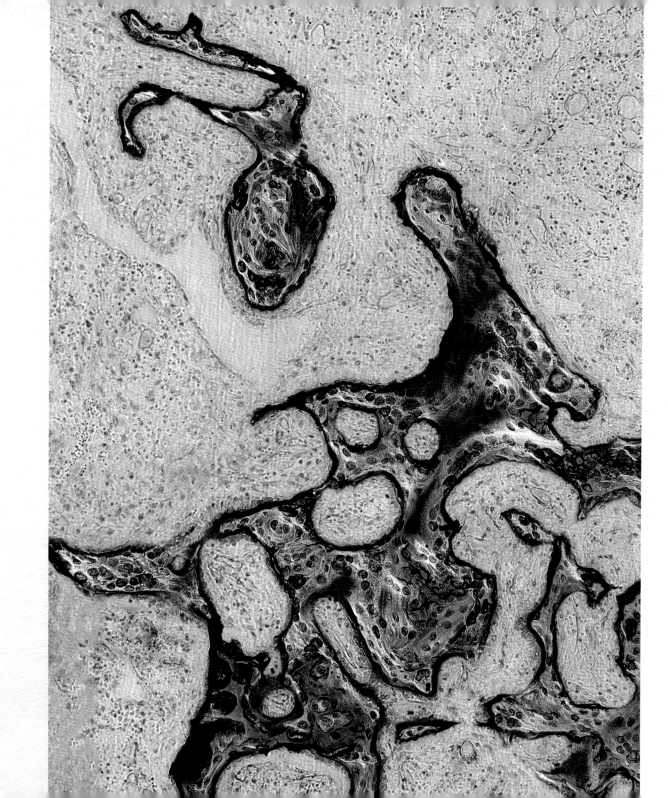

星空 No.9

未脱钙骨组织磨片，X200，明视野 + 偏振光，
2019

Starry sky No.9

Cortical bone, Ground section, X200, Light field
+ polarized light, 2019

林想
梦

梦想

张未晨，9 岁

——

Dream

Zhang Weichen, 9

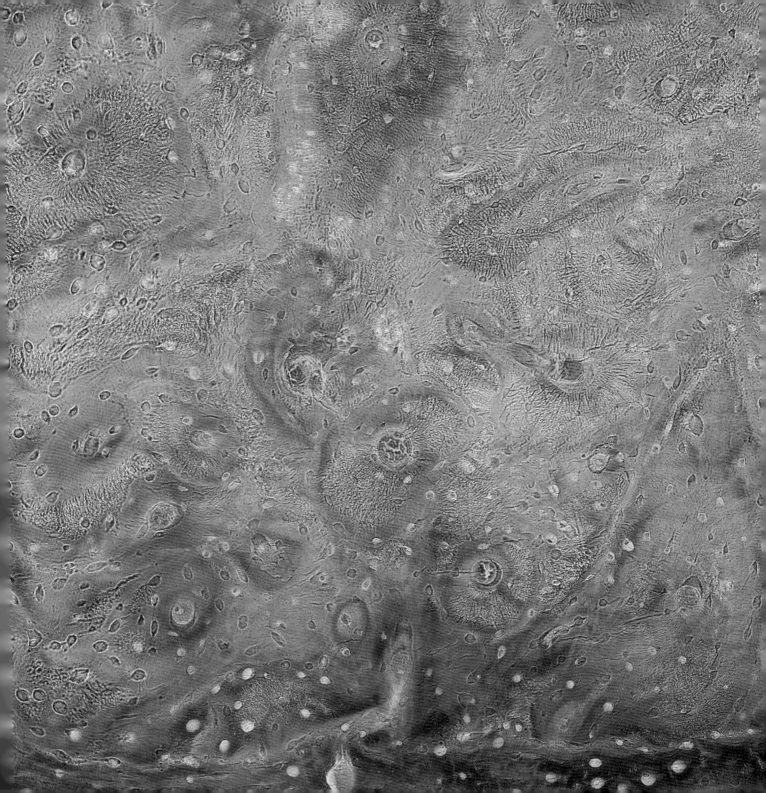

天书 No.110

未脱钙骨组织磨片，X100，偏振光，2019

Heavenly script No.110

Cortical bone, Ground section, X100, Polarized light, 2019

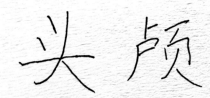

头颅

梁弈澄，10 岁

Skull

Liang Yicheng, 10

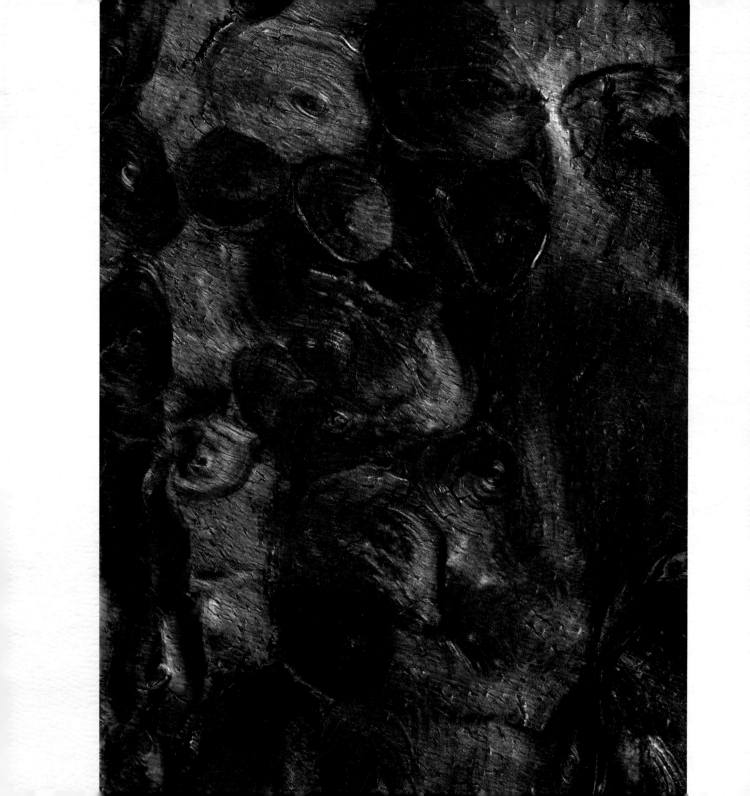

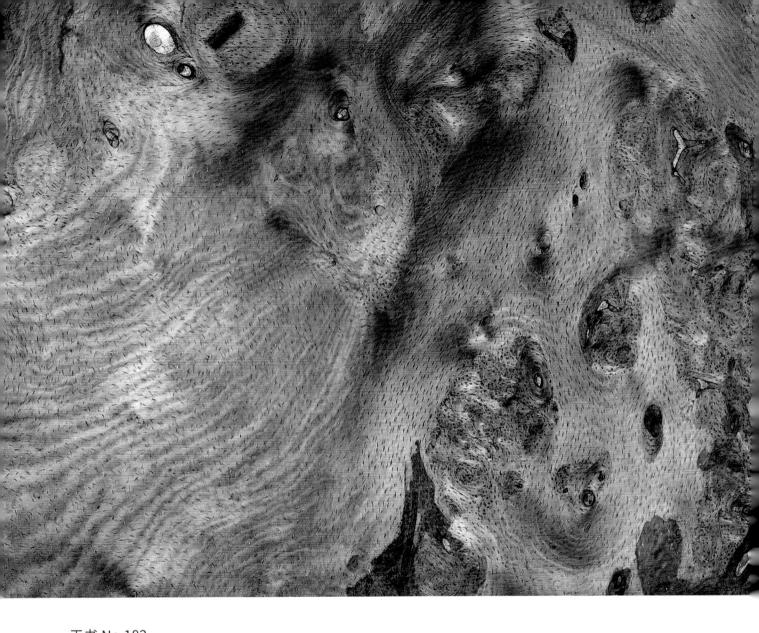

天书 No.182

未脱钙骨组织磨片，X40，明视野 + 偏振光，2021

Heavenly script No.182

Cortical bone, Ground section, X40, Light field + polarized light, 2021

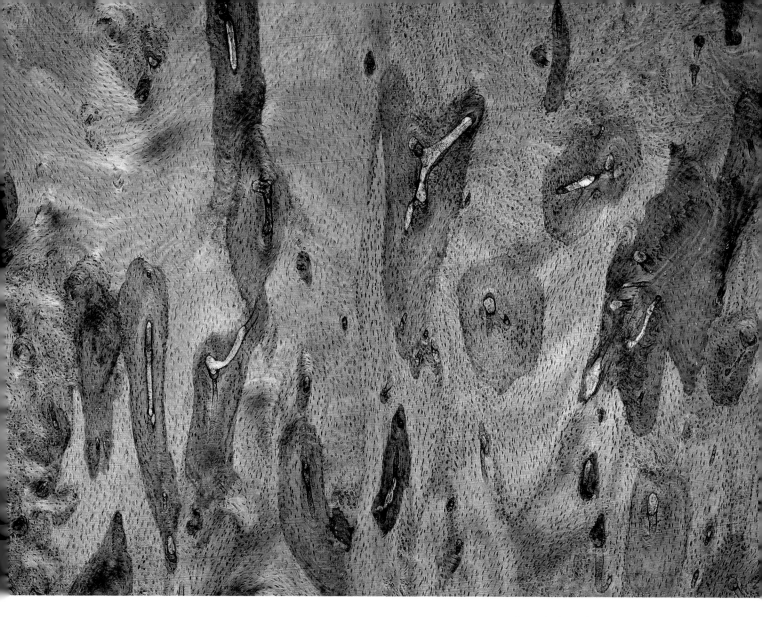

骨骼是 动物的 化石

骨骼是动物的化石

宣子杉，11 岁

Skeleton is an animal's fossil.

Xuan Zishan, 11

凤舞

脱钙骨组织切片，X40，偏振光，2013

Phoenix dance

Trabecular bone, Tissue section, X40, Polarized light, 2013

躯干骨

躯干骨

周语欣，12 岁

Bones of trunk

Zhou Yuxin, 12

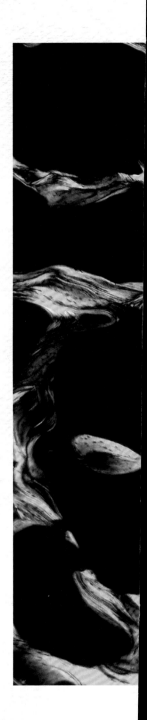

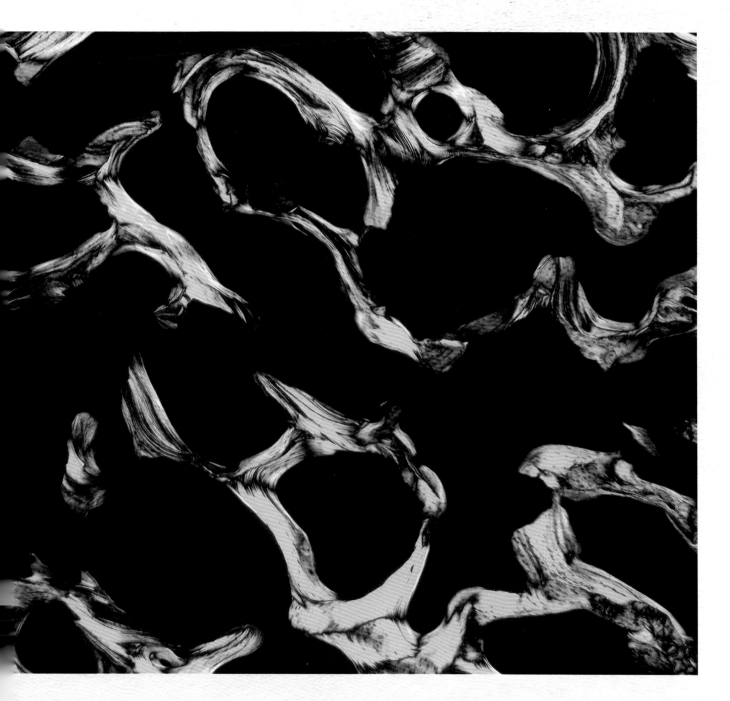

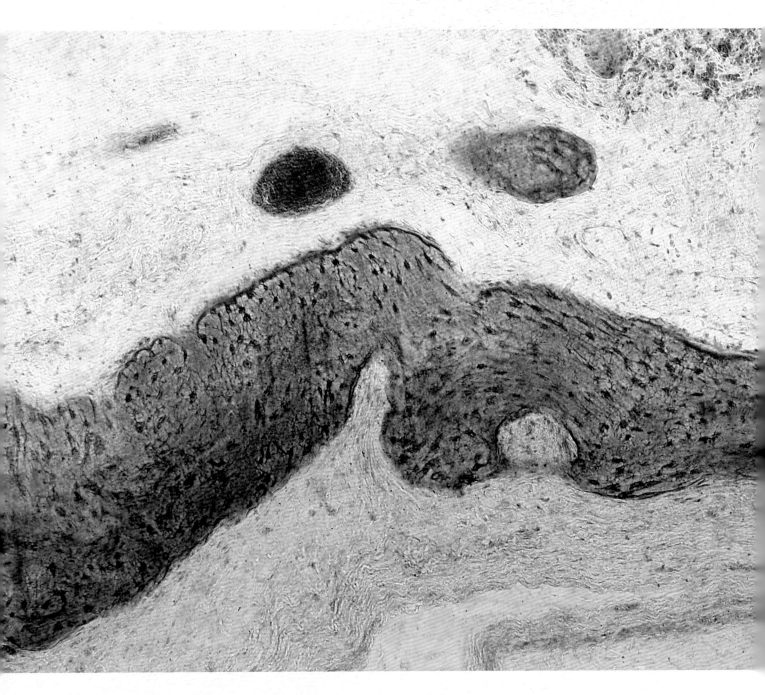

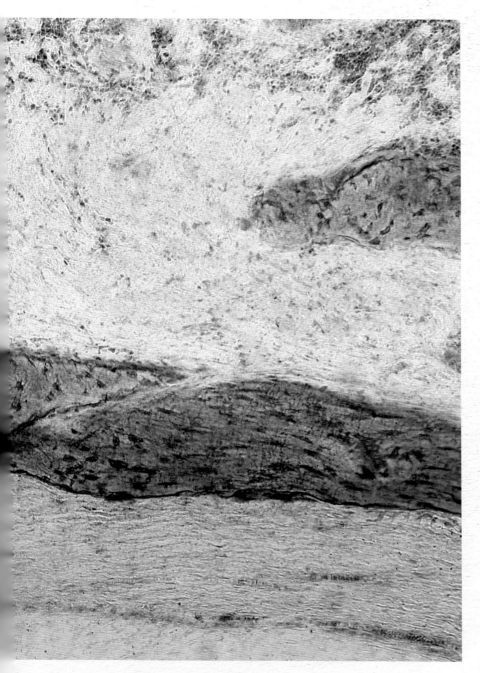

江南

脱钙骨组织切片，X200，明视野，2017

South of the Yangtze River

Trabecular bone, Tissue section, X200,
Light field, 2017

你若精彩，天自安排

你若精彩，天自安排。

王心笛，13 岁

Your splendid performance will
naturally invite the blessing.

Wang Xindi, 13

祭红

脱钙骨组织切片，X100，明视野，2012

Red sacrifice

Cortical bone, Tissue section, X100, Light field, 2012

舞勺之年

舞勺之年

刘佳璐，14 岁

The year of learning to dance the ko (of the duke of Zhou)

Liu Jialu, 14

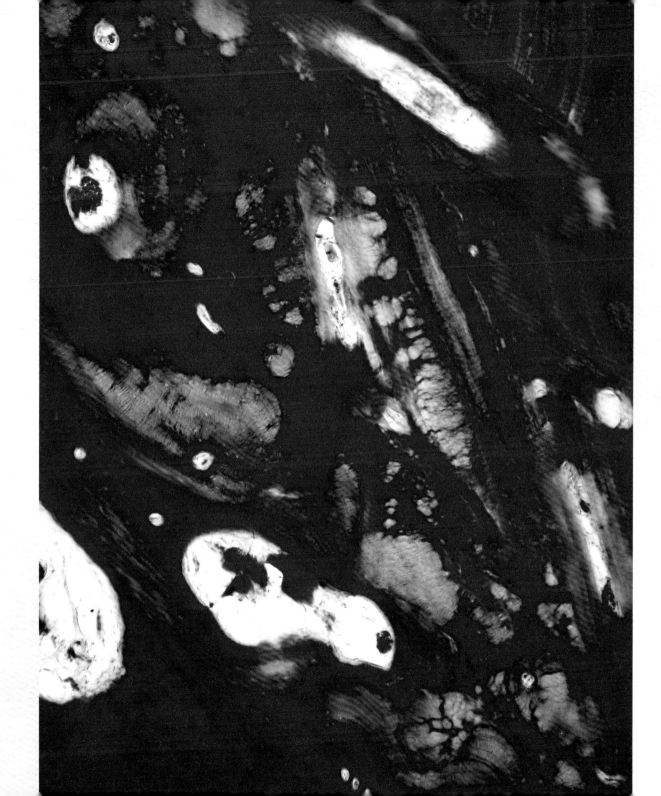

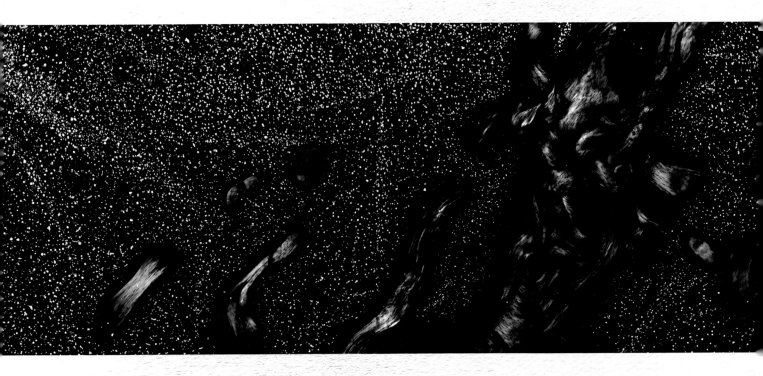

星辰

脱钙骨组织切片，X40，偏振光，2017

Stars

Trabecular bone, Tissue section, X40, Polarized light, 2017

时间带我们穿越

时间带我们穿越

刘鼎奇，15 岁

Time takes us through a space-time continuum.

Liu Dingqi, 15

手稿 No.2

未脱钙骨关节组织磨片，X12.5，明视野 + 偏振光，2019

Manuscript No.2

Bone and joint, Ground section, X12.5, Light field + polarized light, 2019

成长的痕迹

成长的痕迹

梁子舒，16 岁

The trace of growing up

Liang Zishu, 16

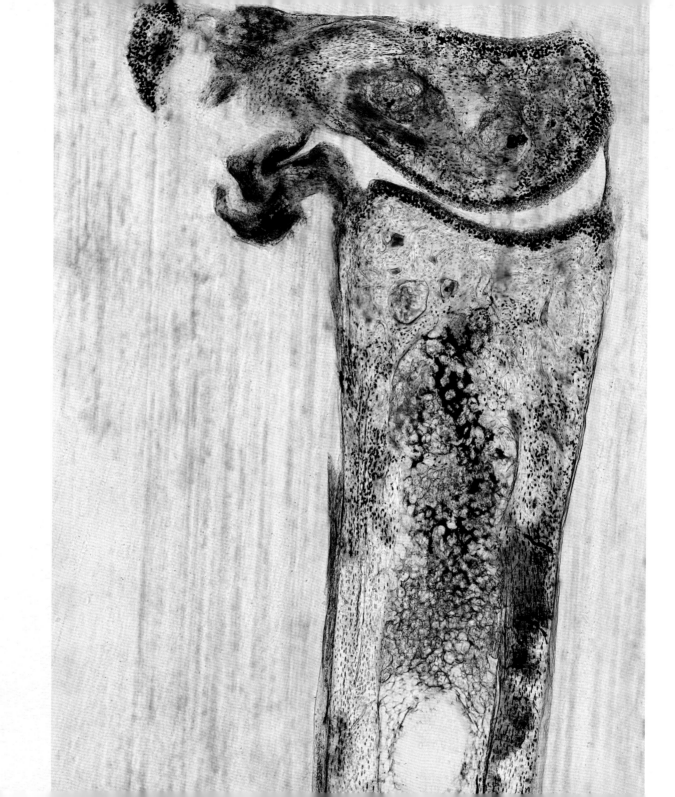

长袖 No.2

未脱钙骨组织磨片，X40，明视野 + 偏振光，2020

Long sleeve No.2

Trabecular bone, Ground section, X40, Light field + polarized light, 2020

恰同学少年

恰同学少年

彭湃风，17 岁

Just when we were young

Peng Paifeng, 17

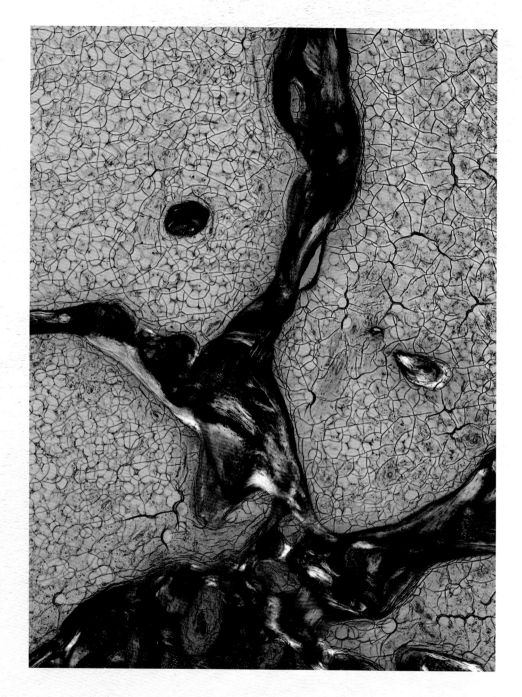

蓝色狂想

未脱钙骨组织及封片胶磨片，X40，明视野 + 偏振光，2020

Blue fantasy

Cortical bone and sealing gel, Ground section, X40, Light field + polarized light, 2020

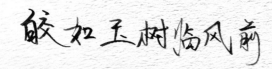

皎如玉树临风前

冯诗淇，18 岁

A jade tree stands in the wind.

Feng Shiqi, 18

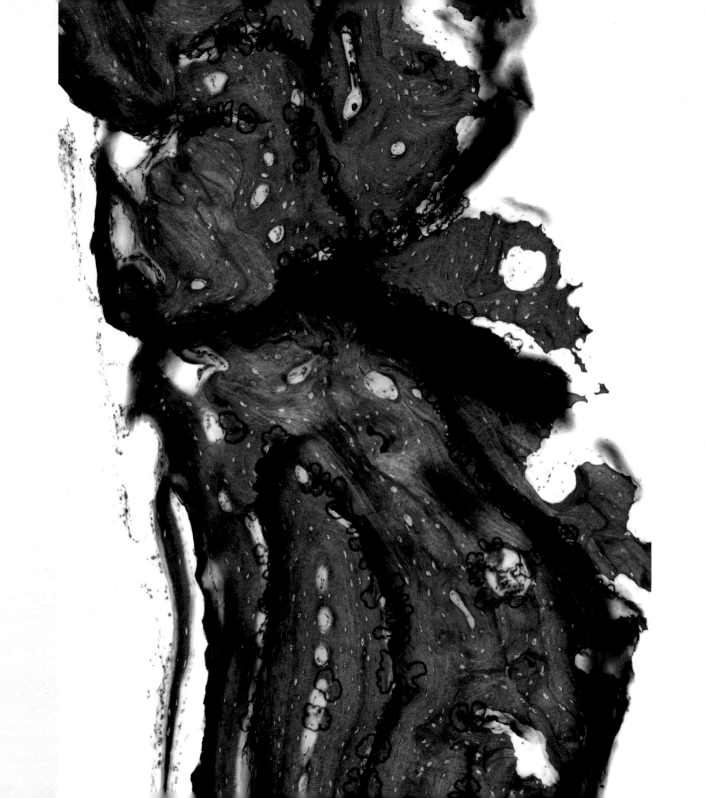

天书 No.55

脱钙骨组织切片，X100，偏振光，2014

Heavenly script No.55

Trabecular bone, Tissue section, X100, Polarized light, 2014

秀骨

杨睿思，19 岁，大学生

The graceful bone

Yang Ruisi, 19, University student

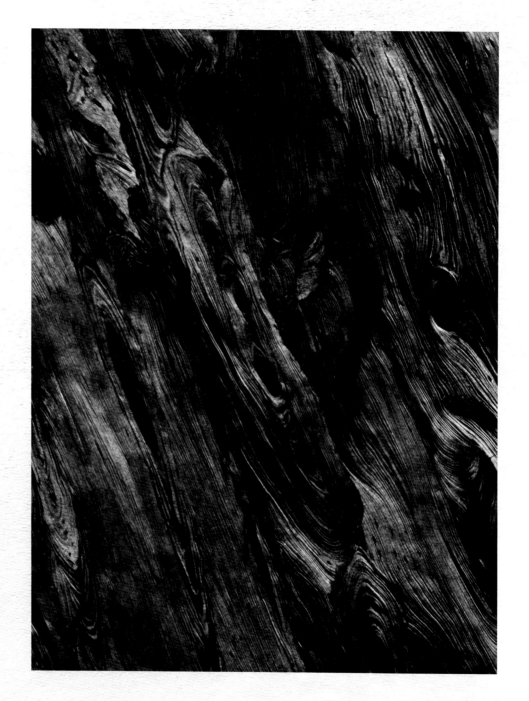

红蘑菇

脱钙骨组织切片，X12.5，明视野，2012

Red mushroom

Cortical and trabecular bone, Tissue section, X12.5, Light field, 2012

你若盛开，蝴蝶自来。

你若盛开，蝴蝶自来。

魏巧冉，20 岁，实习口腔护士

If you bloom, the butterfly will come.

Wei Qiaoran, 20, Dental nurse intern

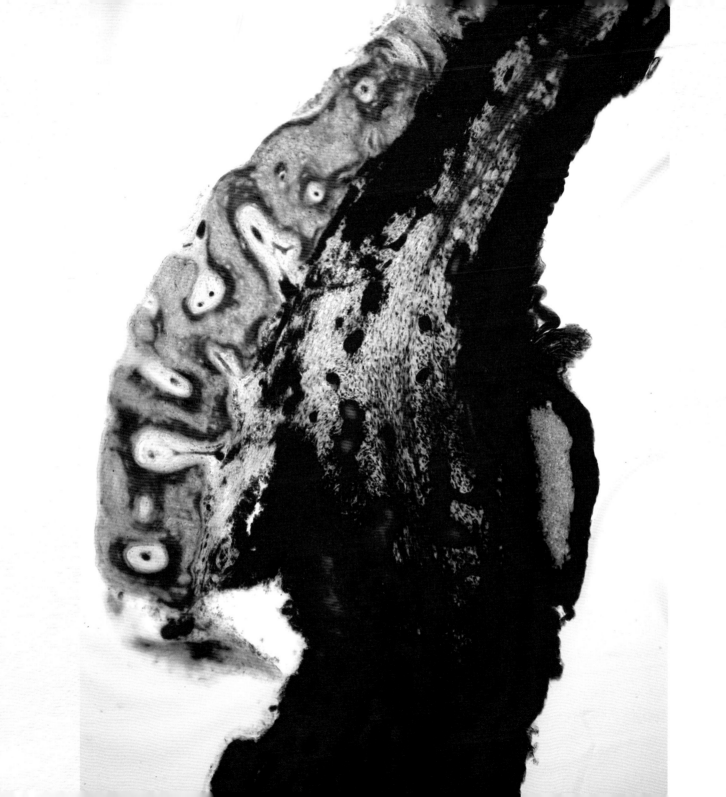

甲骨文 No.1

脱钙骨组织切片，X40，明视野，2015

Oracle No.1

Trabecular bone, Tissue section, X40, Light field, 2015

柳骨

刘文卉，21 岁，护士

Liu style calligraphy

Liu Wenhui, 21, Nurse

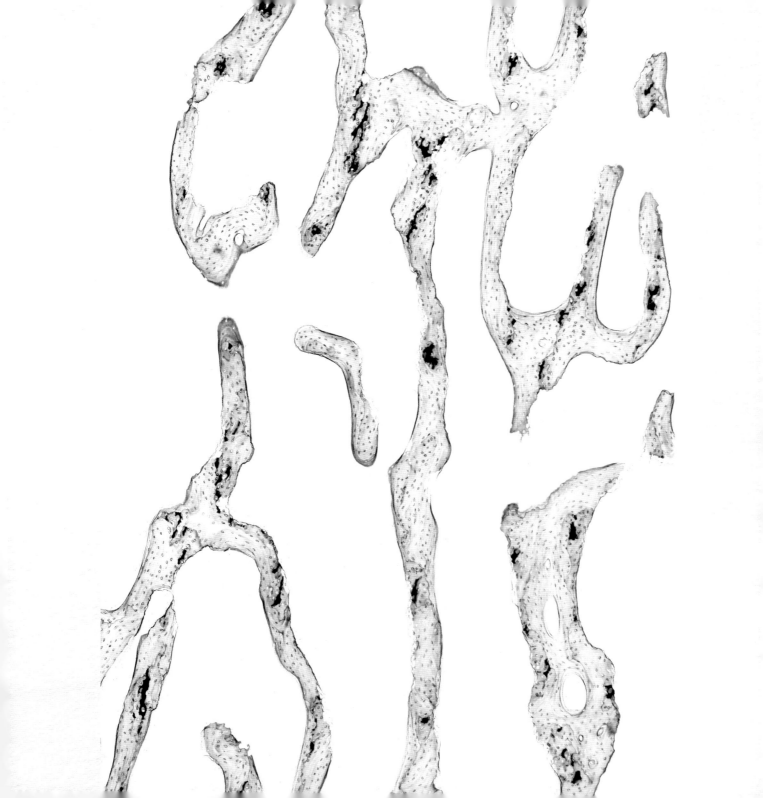

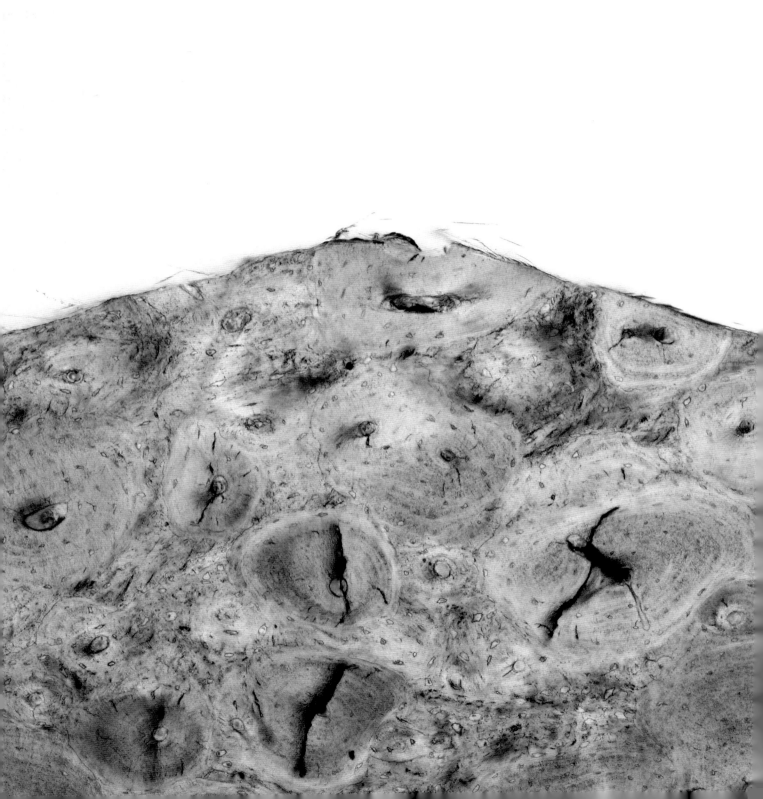

前山

未脱钙骨组织磨片，X100，明视野，2013

Front mountain

Cortical bone, Ground section, X100, Light field, 2013

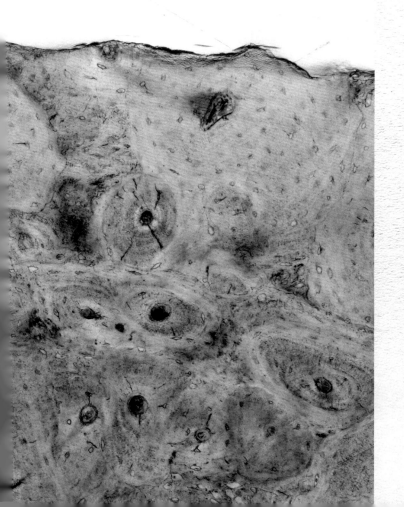

道骨仙风，冰清玉洁。

常嘉迪，22 岁，大学生

The demeanor of bone is as clean as ice and as pure as jade.

Chang Jiadi, 22, University student

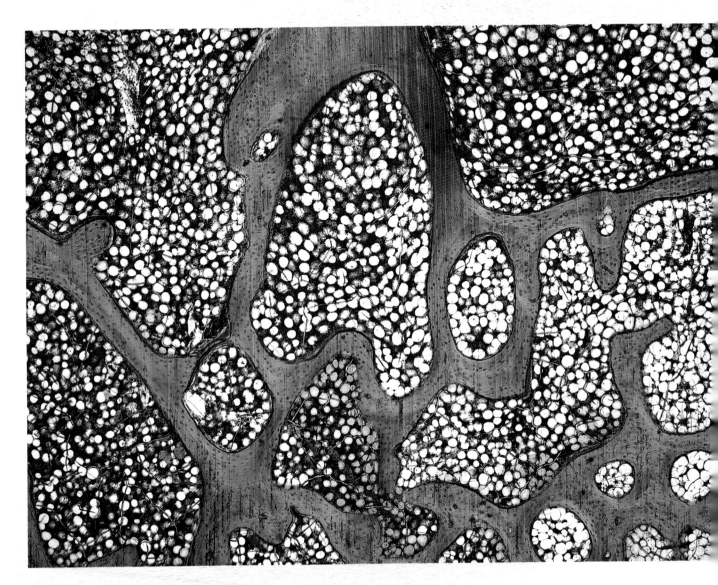

绿植类

未脱钙骨组织磨片，X40，明视野，2021

Green plants

Trabecular bone, Ground section, X40, Light field, 2021

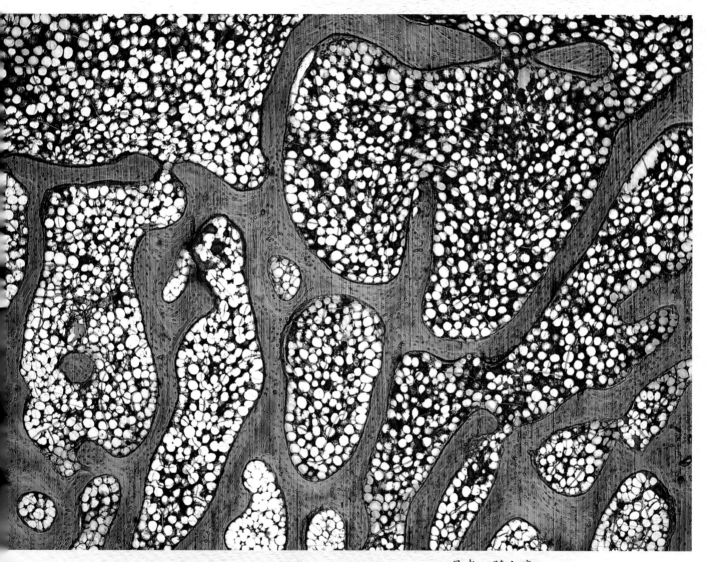

骨者，髓之府。

石闪闪，23 岁，护士

Bone houses and nurtures its marrow.

Shi Shanshan, 23, Nurse

骨者，髓之府

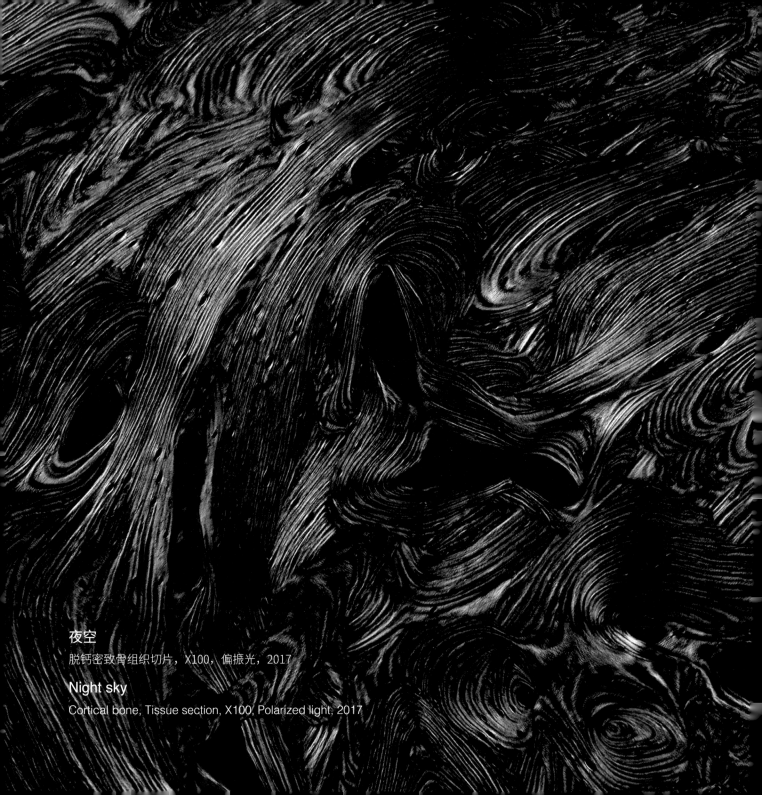

夜空

脱钙密致骨组织切片，X100，偏振光，2017

Night sky

Cortical bone, Tissue section, X100, Polarized light, 2017

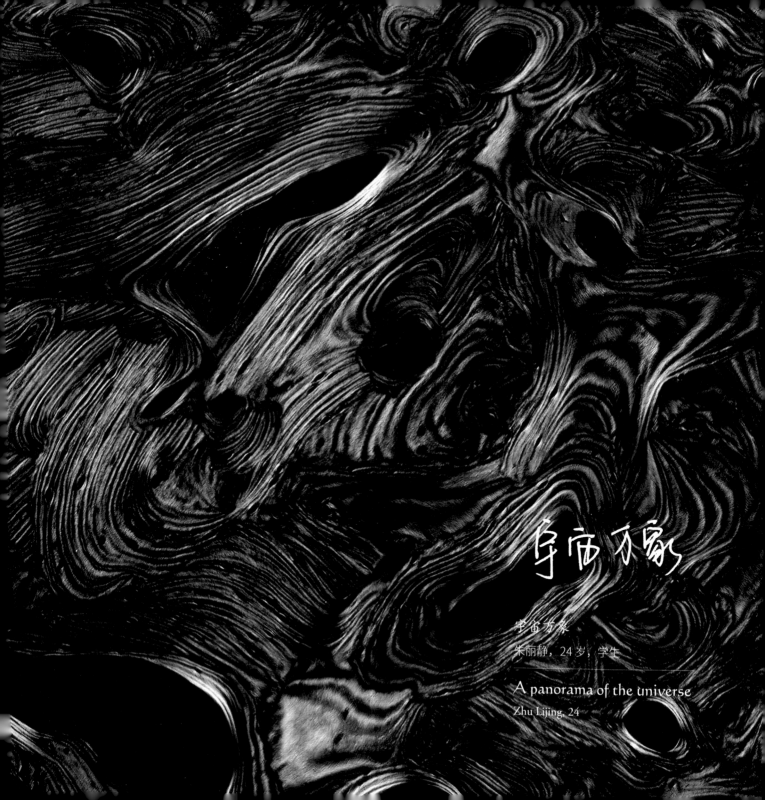

宇宙万象

朱丽静，24 岁，学生

A panorama of the universe
Zhu Lijing, 24

蒙古舞

未脱钙骨组织磨片，X40，明视野 + 偏振光，2020

Mongolian dance

Trabecular bone, Ground section, X40, Light field +
polarized light, 2020

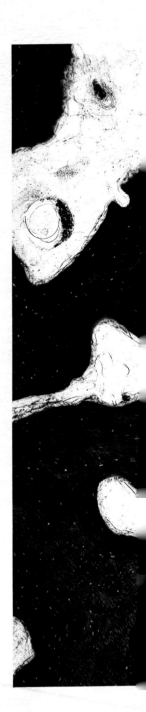

拙朴浑厚

拙朴浑厚

拙朴浑厚

张嘉欣，25 岁，护士
王海侠，25 岁，护士

Vigorous simplicity and honesty

Zhang Jiaxin, 25, Nurse

Wang Haixia, 25, Nurse

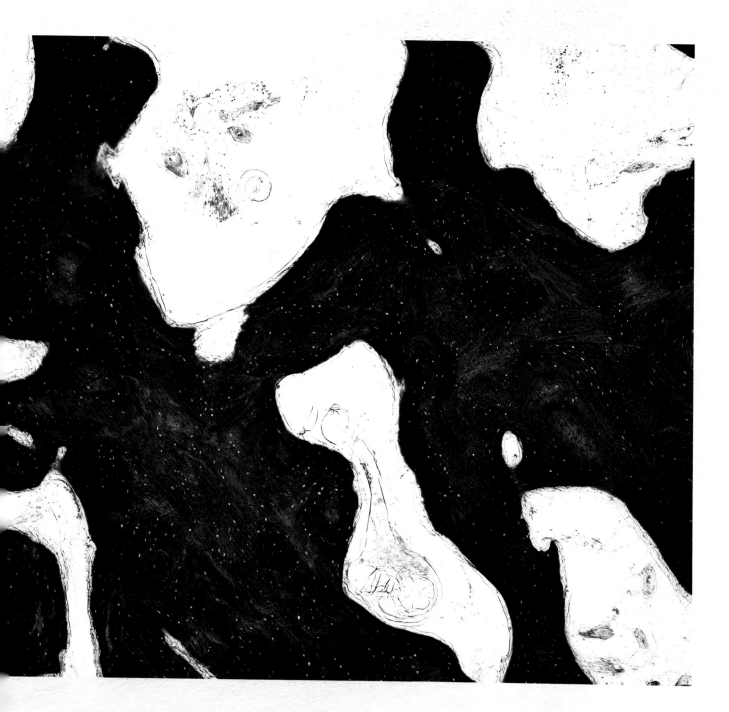

魅影

脱钙骨组织切片，X40，偏振光，2016

Phantom

Bone and soft tissues, Tissue section, X40, Polarized light, 2016

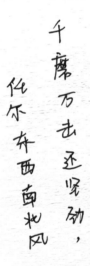

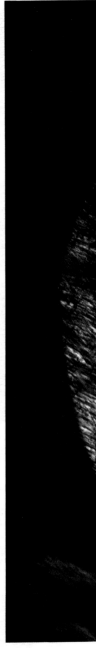

千磨万击还坚劲，任尔东西南北风。

王珊，26 岁，研究生

Whatever tribulations may strike, I remain strong and undaunted.

Wang Shan, 26, Graduate student

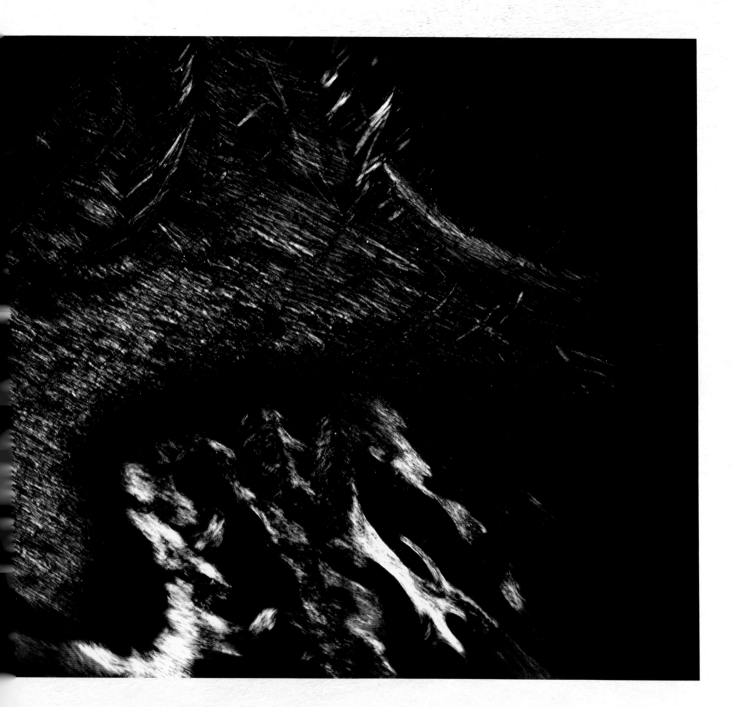

骨折

脱钙骨组织切片（切片部分折损），X100，明视野，2011

Bone fracture

Trabecular bone, Tissue section (slide partly broken), X100, Light field, 2011

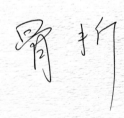

骨折

蔡鑫嘉，27 岁，研究生

Fracture

Cai Xinjia, 27, Graduate student

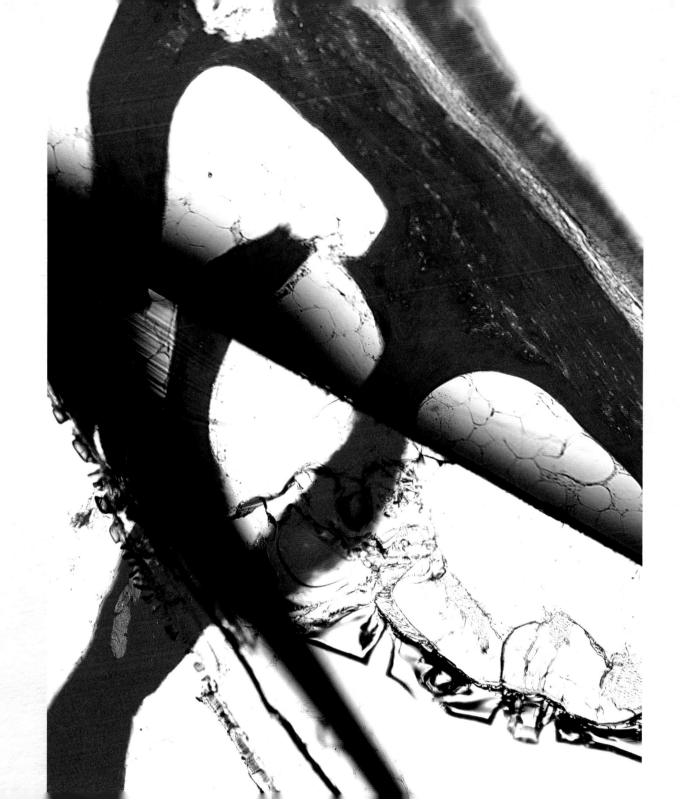

风的颜色

未脱钙骨及周围组织磨片，X40，明视野＋偏振光，2019

The colors of the wind

Bone and surrounding tissues, Ground section, X40, Light field + polarized light, 2019

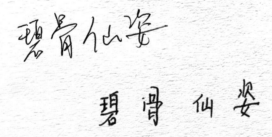

碧骨仙姿

汪鑫，28 岁，口腔医生

刘晓筱，28 岁，研究生

Fairy-like beauty in jade-like bone

Wang Xin, 28, Dentist

Liu Xiaoxiao, 28, Graduate student

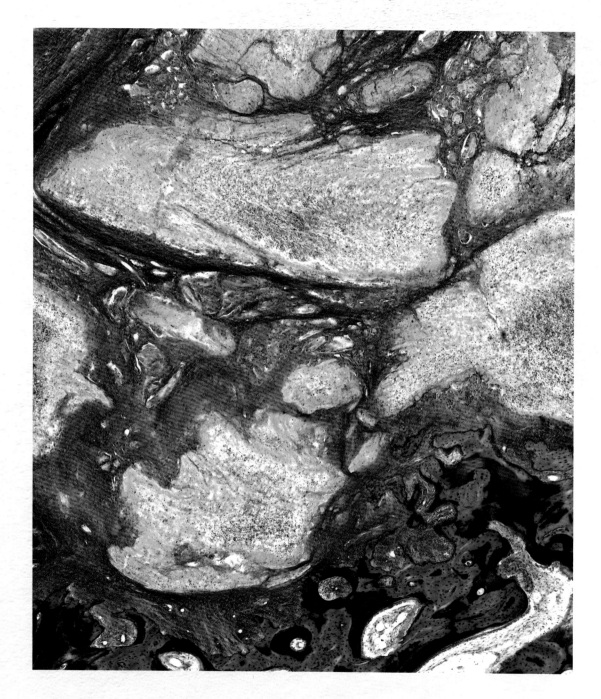

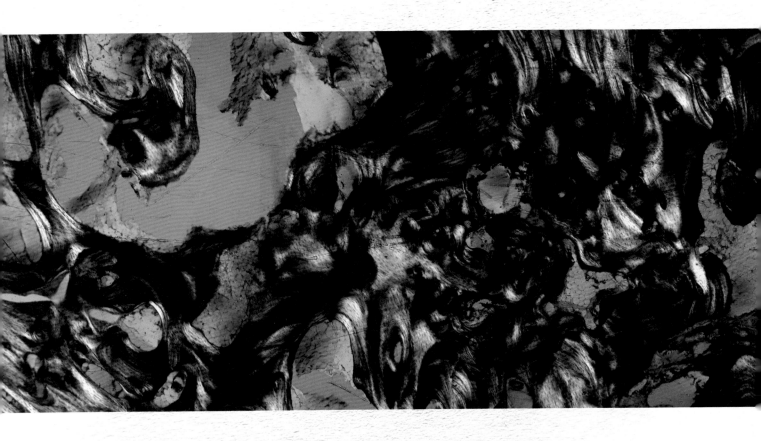

风骨 No.47

脱钙骨组织切片，X40，明视野 + 偏振光，2017

Backbone No.47

Cortical and trabecular bone, Tissue section, X40, Light field + polarized light, 2017

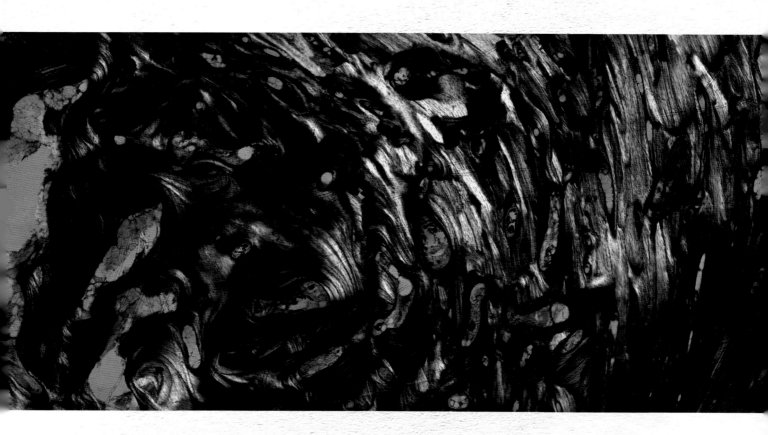

笔迹者，界也；流美者，人也。

笔迹者，界也；流美者，人也。

张奥博，29 岁，研究生

Handwriting is just a recorded mark, but its real beauty lies in the ultimate pursuit of art.

Zhang Aobo, 29, Graduate student

风骨 No.8

脱钙骨组织切片，X100，偏振光，2013

Backbone No.8

Trabecular bone, Tissue section, X100, Polarized light, 2013

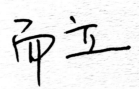

而立

张晔，30 岁，研究生

Man establishes himself at thirty.

Zhang Ye, 30, Graduate student

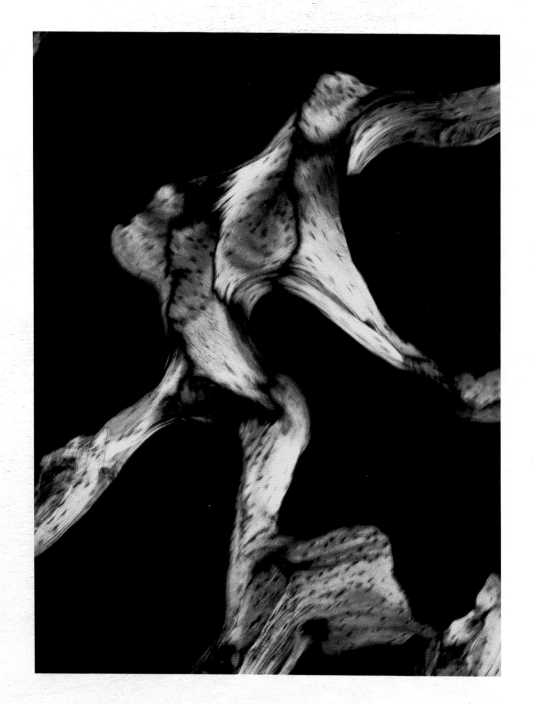

风骨 No.37

脱钙骨组织切片，X100，明视野，2016

Backbone No.37

Trabecular bone, Tissue section, X100, Light field, 2016

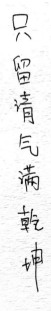

只留清气满乾坤

李冬遥，31岁，工程师

(The plum flowers') delicate fragrance lingers in the air seeking no fame.

Li Dongyao, 31, Engineer

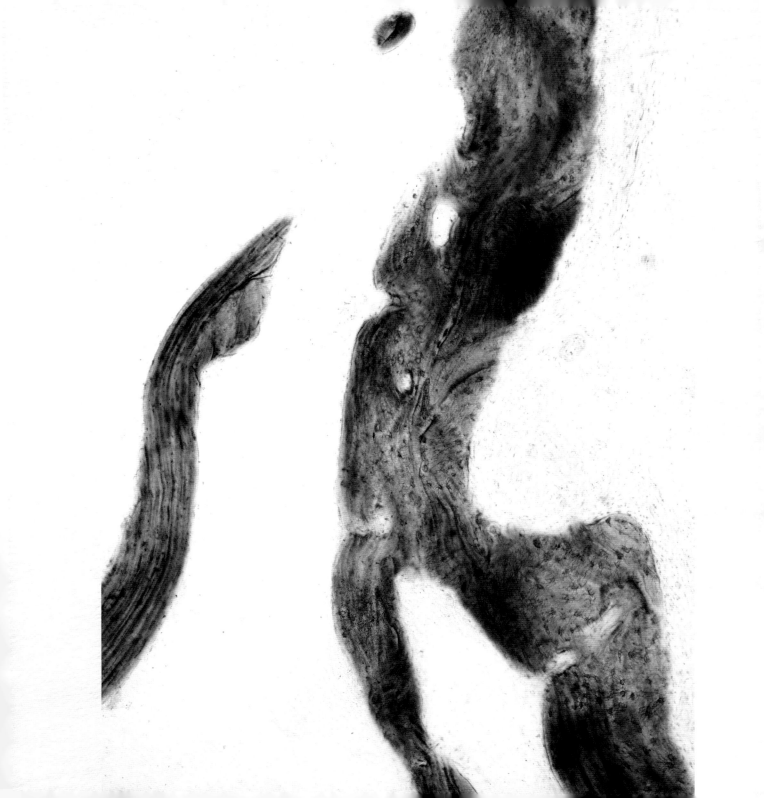

风骨 No.12

脱钙骨组织切片，X100，明视野＋偏振光，2013

Backbone No.12

Trabecular bone, Tissue section, X100, Light field + polarized light, 2013

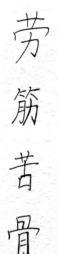

劳筋苦骨

蔡青青，32岁，医务人员

To toughen the muscle and bone

Cai Qingqing, 32, Medical staff

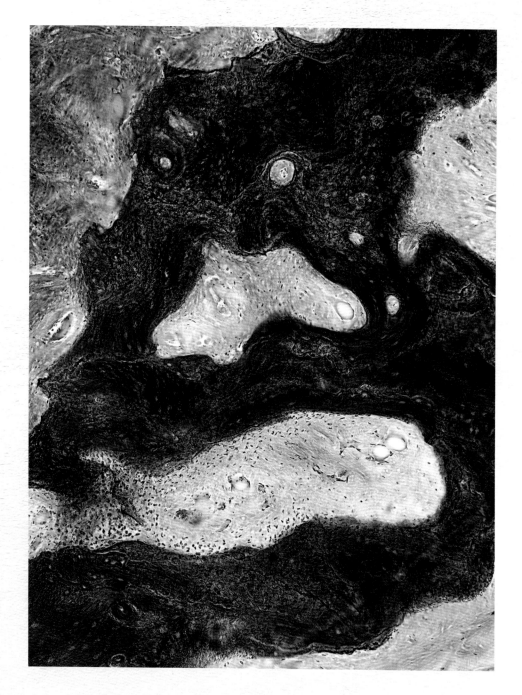

一撇

脱钙骨组织切片，X40，偏振光，2019

One stroke

Trabecular bone, Tissues section, X40, Polarized light, 2019

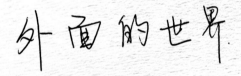

外面的世界

张滢，33 岁，工程师

The outside world

Zhang Ying, 33, Engineer

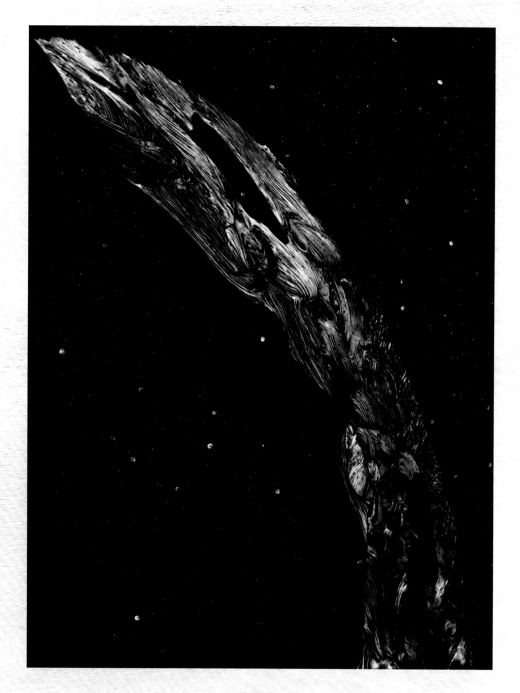

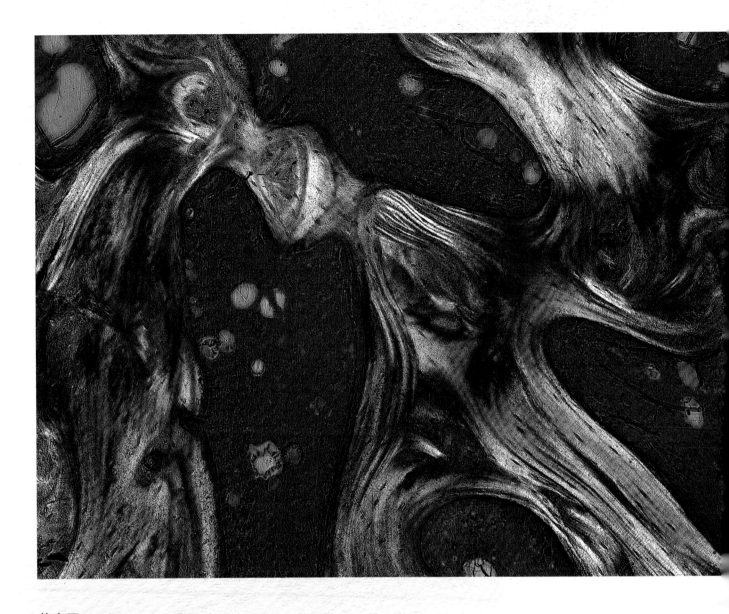

黄金甲 No.1

未脱钙骨组织磨片，X100，明视野 + 偏振光，2019

Golden armor No.1

Trabecular bone, Ground section, X100, Light field + polarized light, 2019

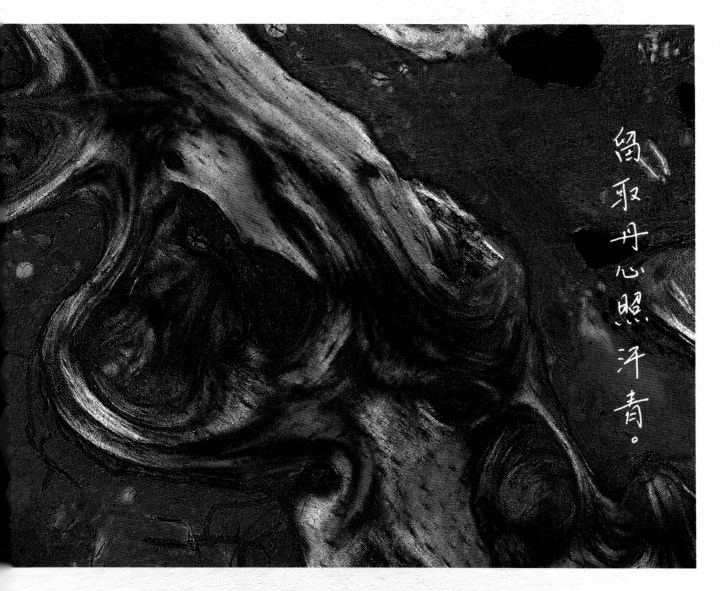

留取丹心照汗青

留取丹心照汗青

洪瑛瑛，34 岁，口腔医生

My loyalty to the motherland is worthy of a page in history.

Hong Yingying, 34, Dentist

天书 No.145
未脱钙骨组织磨片，X40， 偏振光，2020

Heavenly script No.145
Trabecular bone, Ground section, X40, Polarized light, 2020

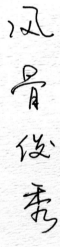

风骨俊秀

杨静文，35 岁，口腔医生

Elegant bone of integrity

Yang Jingwen, 35, Dentist

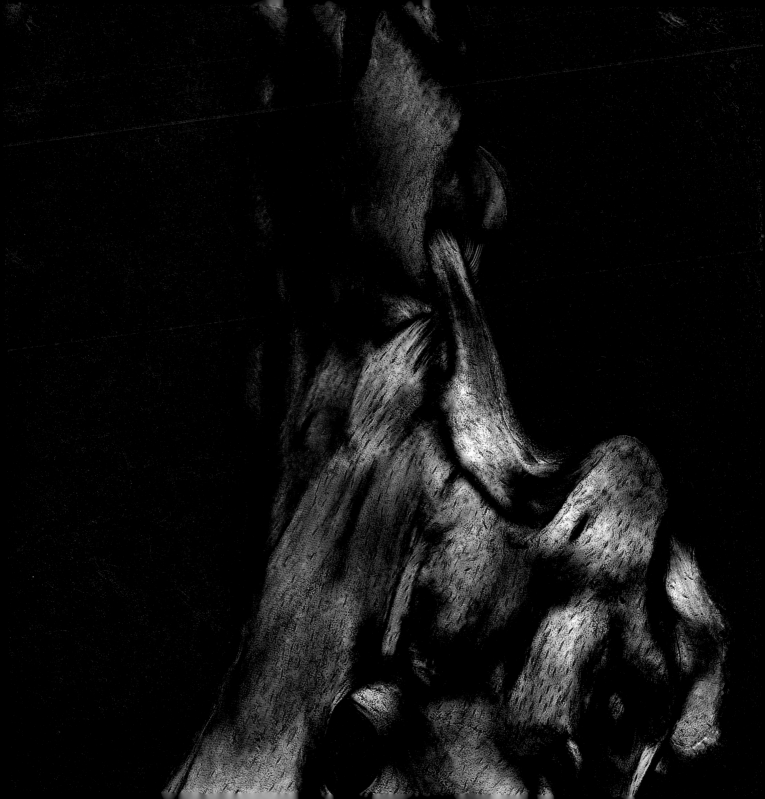

天书 No.98

未脱钙骨组织磨片，X100，明视野 + 偏振光，2019

Heavenly script No.98

Trabecular bone, Ground section, X100, Light field + polarized light, 2019

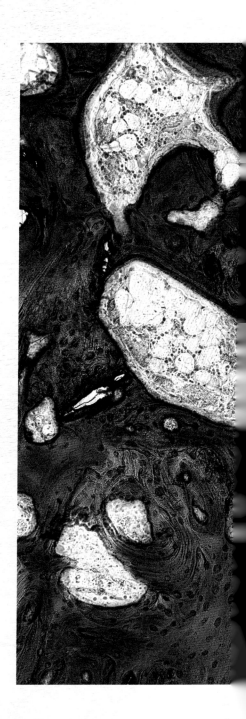

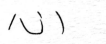

心画

黄金，36 岁，企业管理人员

Painting in the heart

Huang Jin, 36, Enterprise manager

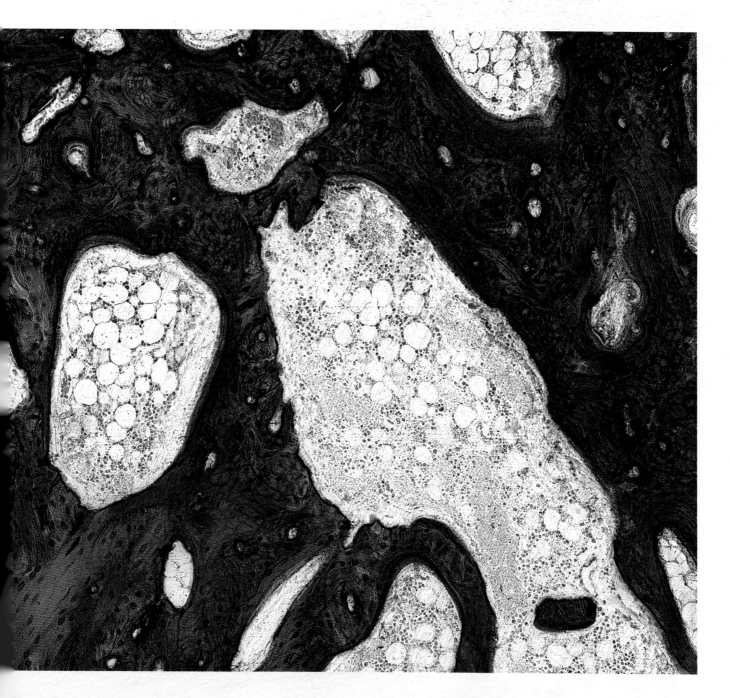

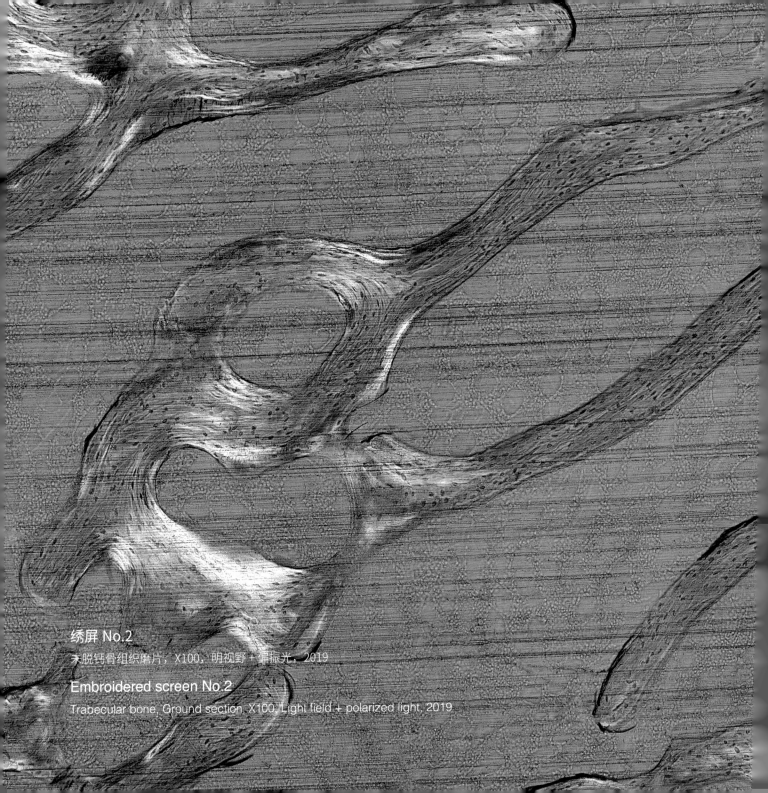

绣屏 No.2

未脱钙骨组织磨片，X100，明视野＋偏振光，2019

Embroidered screen No.2

Trabecular bone, Ground section, X100, Light field + polarized light, 2019

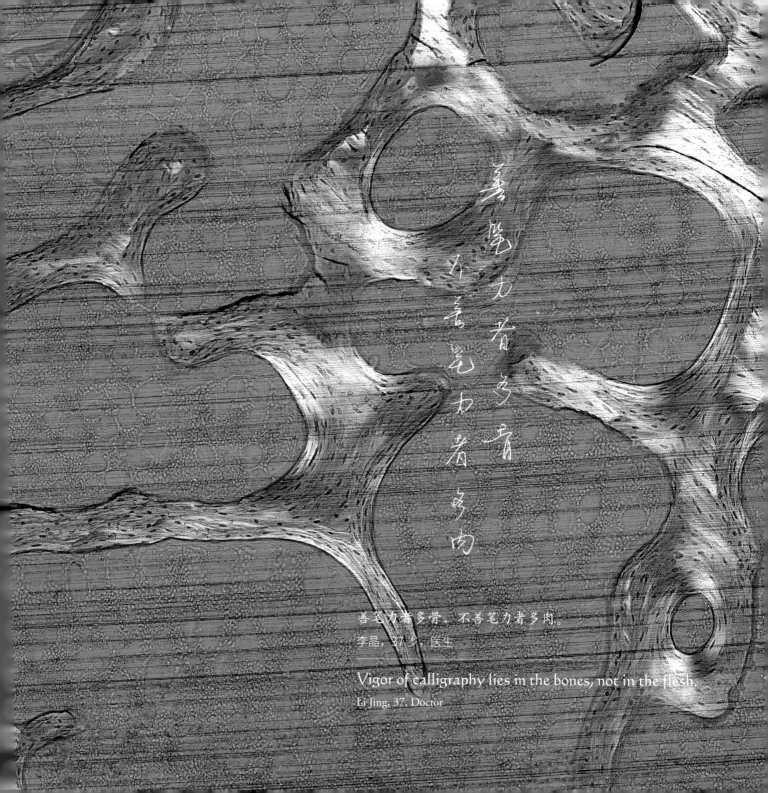

善笔力者多骨，不善笔力者多肉。

李晶，37 岁，医生

Vigor of calligraphy lies in the bones, not in the flesh.

Li Jing, 37, Doctor

天书 No.212

未脱钙骨组织磨片，X40，明视野 + 偏振光，2021

Heavenly script No.212

Cortical bone, Ground section, X40, Light field + polarized light, 2021

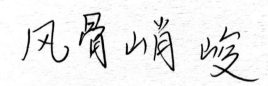

风骨峭峻

司马梓涵，38 岁，口腔医生

A lofty mountain of bone

Sima Zihan, 38, Dentist

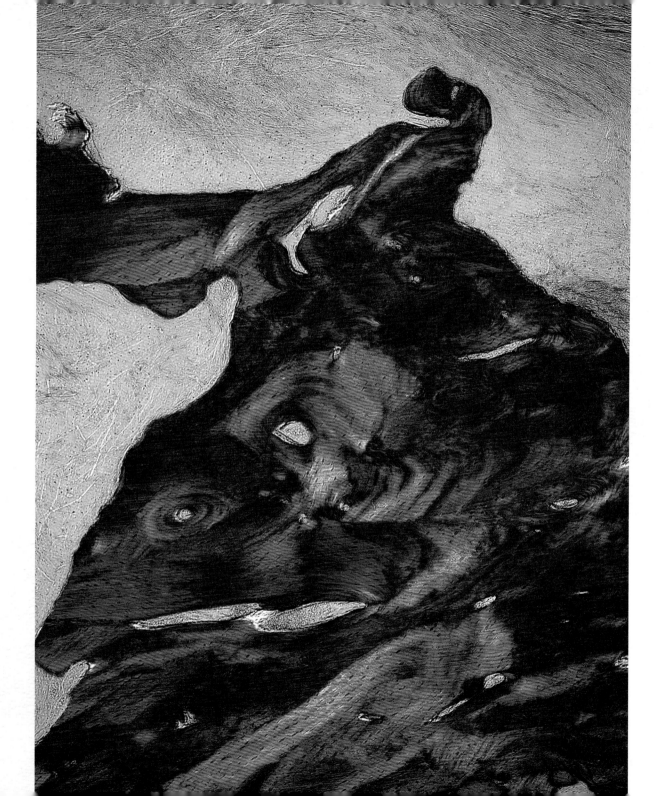

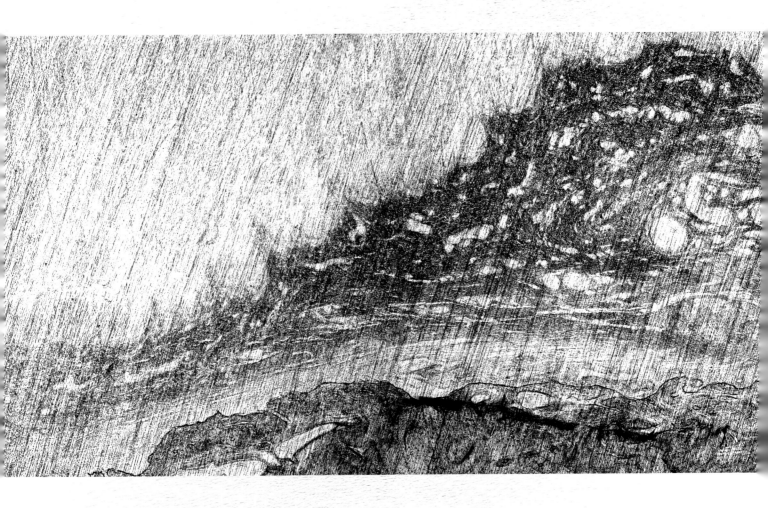

天书 No.210

未脱钙骨及周围软组织磨片，X40，明视野，2021

Heavenly script No.210

Cortical bone and soft tissues, Ground section, X40, Light field, 2021

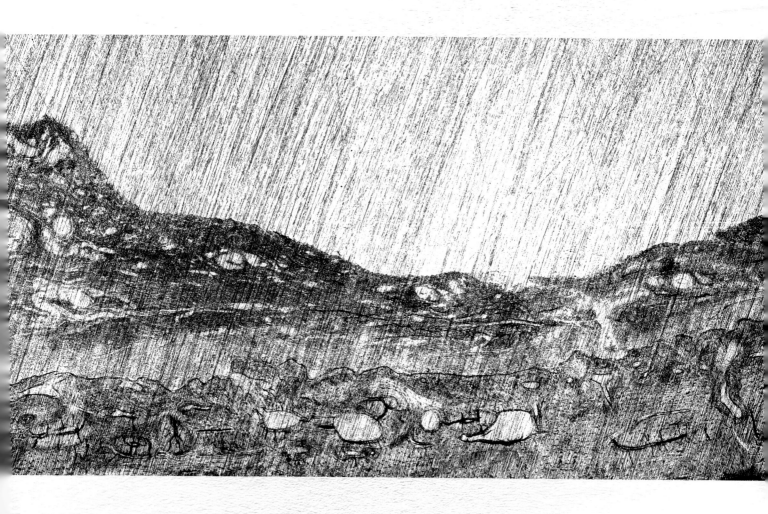

不要人夸好颜色

不要人夸好颜色

刘燕，39 岁，教授

No color is good color.

Liu Yan, 39, Professor

石佛

骨组织未脱钙硬组织切片，X100，明视野，2013

Stone Buddha

Cortical bone, Ground section, X100, Light field, 2013

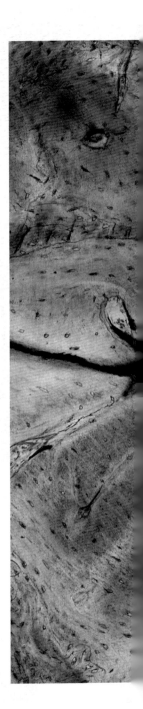

对面不知人有骨

对面不知人有骨

翟洁梅，40 岁，副教授

孙志鹏，40 岁，教授

You could hardly see the bone behind the face.

Zhai Jiemei, 40, Associate professor

Sun Zhipeng, 40, Professor

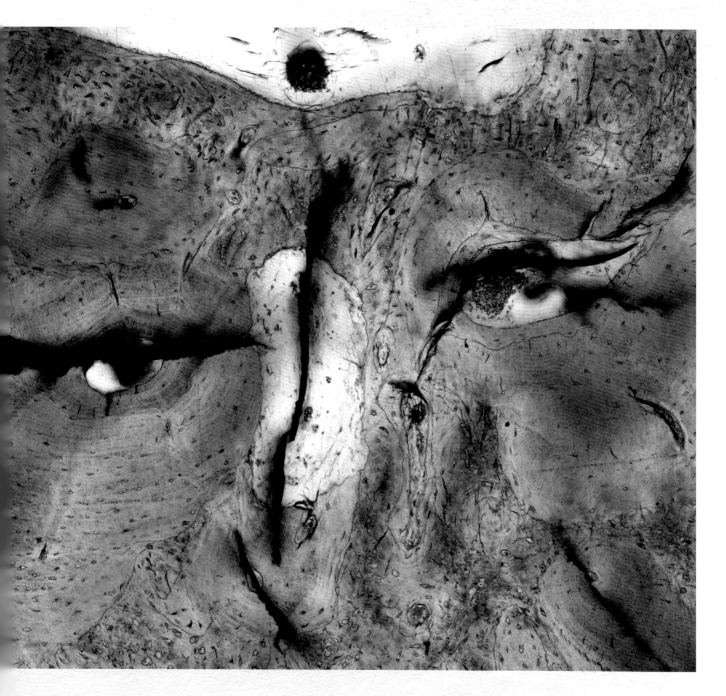

風骨 No.6

脱钙骨组织切片，X12.5，明视野，2012

Backbone No.6

Trabecular bone, Tissue section, X12.5, Light field, 2012

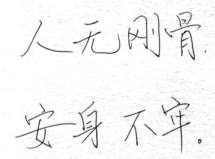

人无刚骨，安身不牢。

张建运，41 岁，副教授

No man is strong without a backbone.

Zhang Jianyun, 41, Associate professor

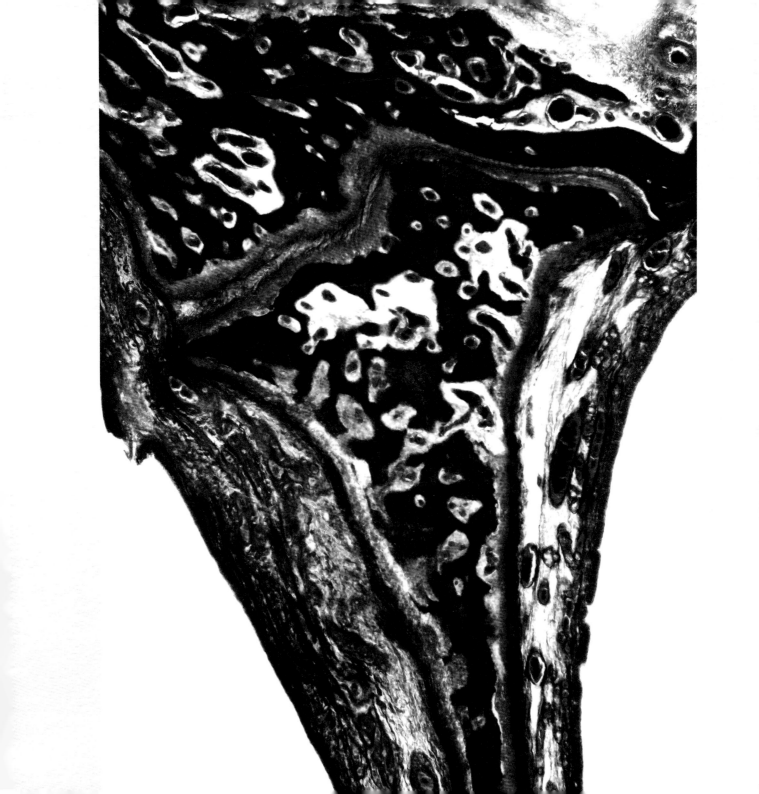

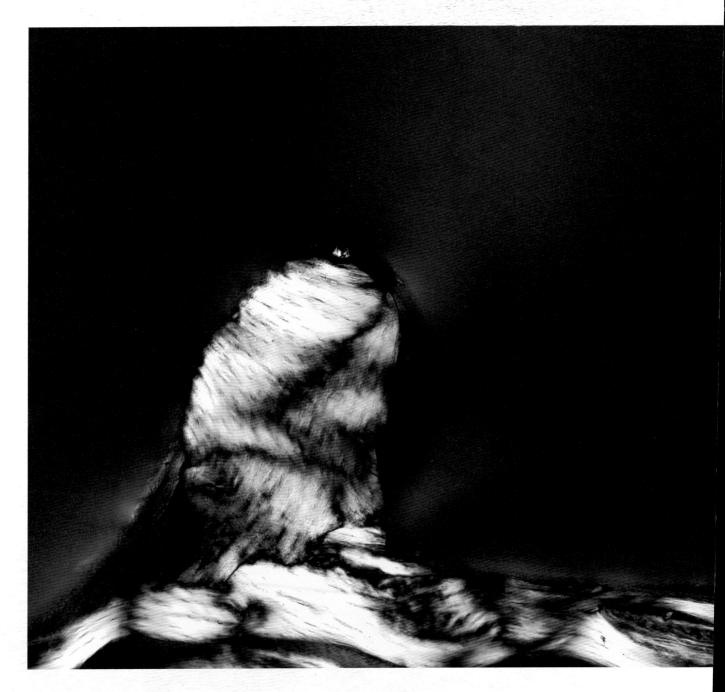

极光

脱钙骨组织切片，X200，偏振光，2013

Aurora

Trabecular bone, Tissue section X200, Polarized light, 2013

我自横刀向天笑，

去留肝胆两昆仑。

我自横刀向天笑，去留肝胆两昆仑。

孙丽莎，42 岁，副研究员

Smiling with a sword in hand, I look skyward; Leave or stay, my will remains lofty like the majestic mountain.

Sun Lisha, 42, Associate professor

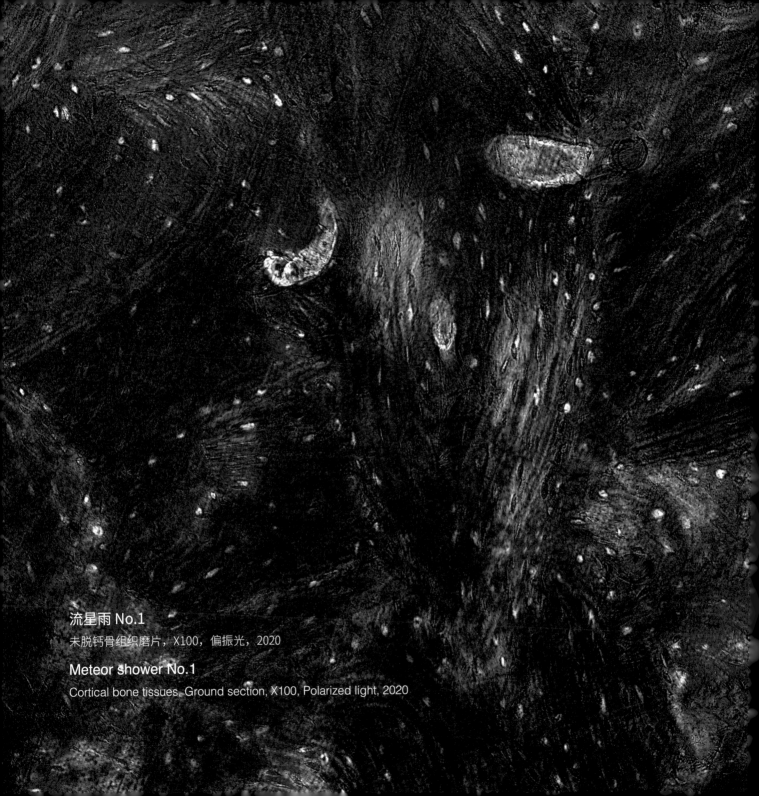

流星雨 No.1

未脱钙骨组织磨片，X100，偏振光，2020

Meteor shower No.1

Cortical bone tissues, Ground section, X100, Polarized light, 2020

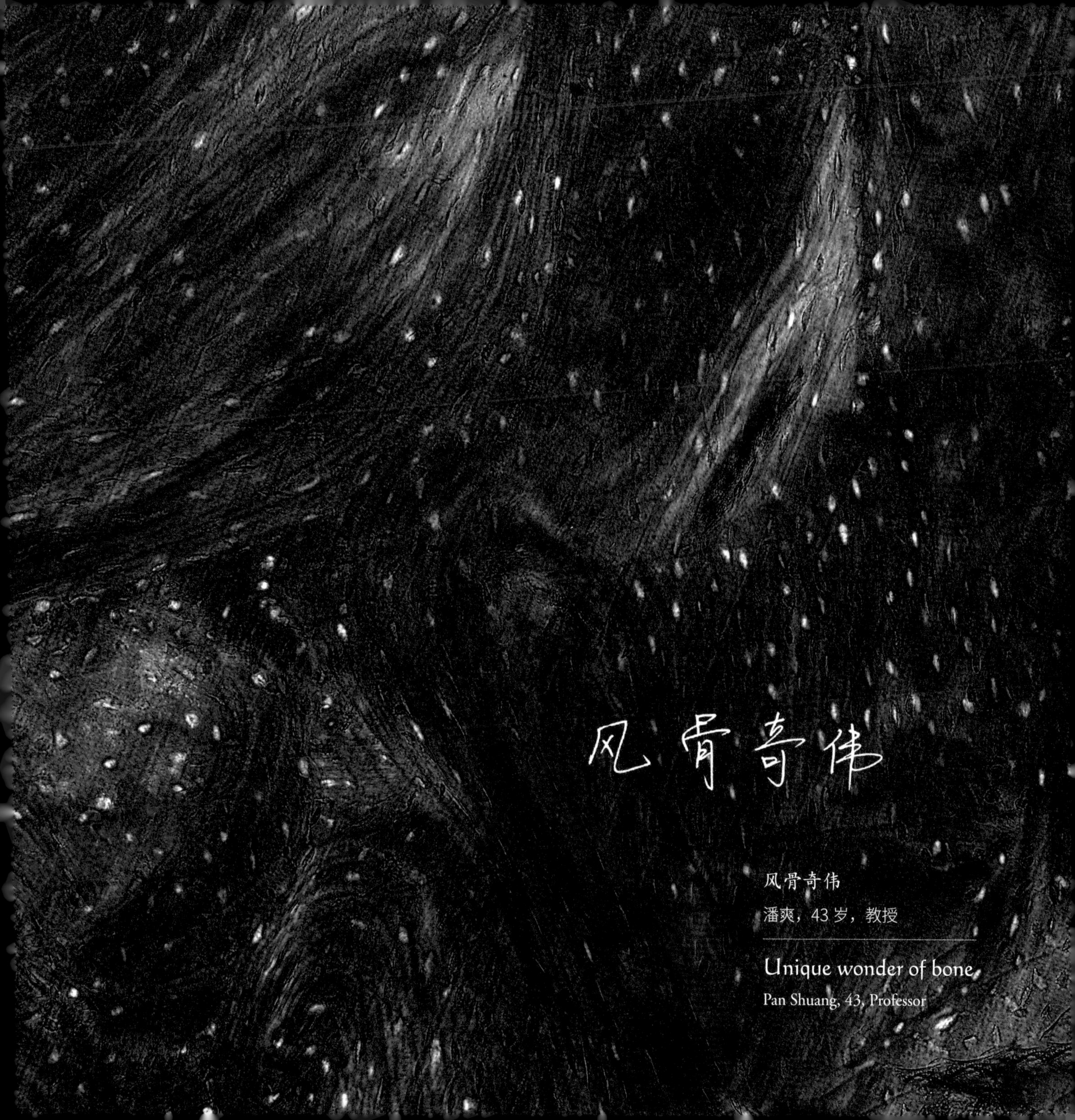

风骨奇伟

风骨奇伟
潘爽，43 岁，教授

Unique wonder of bone
Pan Shuang, 43, Professor

风骨 No.13

脱钙骨组织切片，X200，偏振光，2013

Backbone No.13

Trabecular bone, Tissue section, X200, Polarized light, 2013

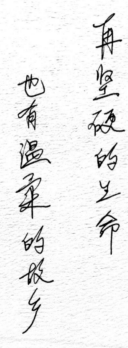

再坚硬的生命也有温柔的故乡

张磊，44 岁，教授

Even the strongest life has its warm cozy home.

Zhang Lei, 44, Professor

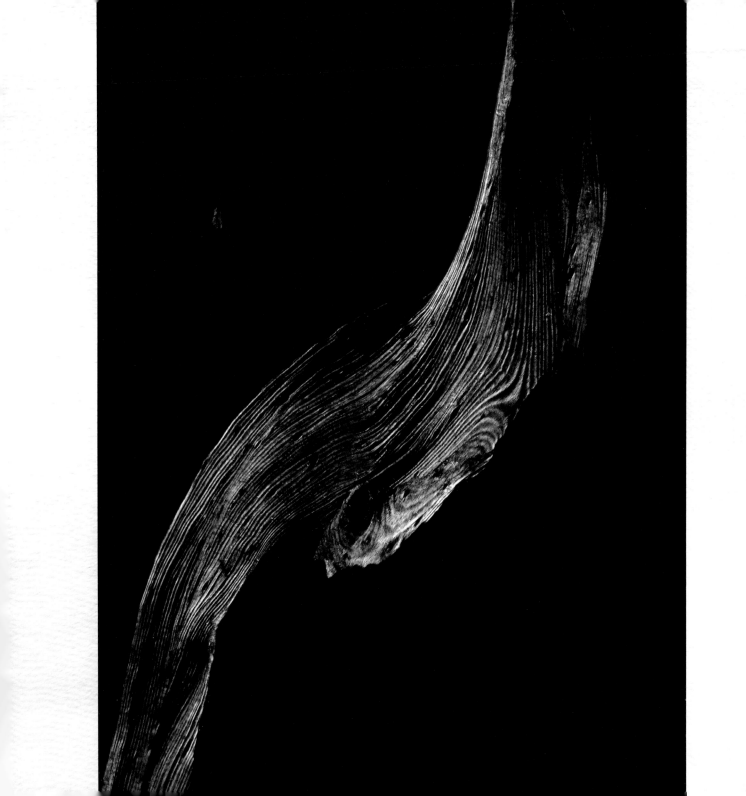

风骨 No.10

未脱钙骨组织磨片，X40，偏振光，2013

Backbone No.10

Trabecular bone, Ground section, X40, Polarized light, 2013

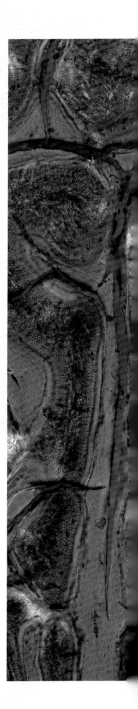

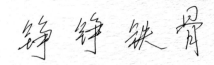

铮铮铁骨

梁炜，45 岁，教授

Bone as hard as iron

Liang Wei, 45, Professor

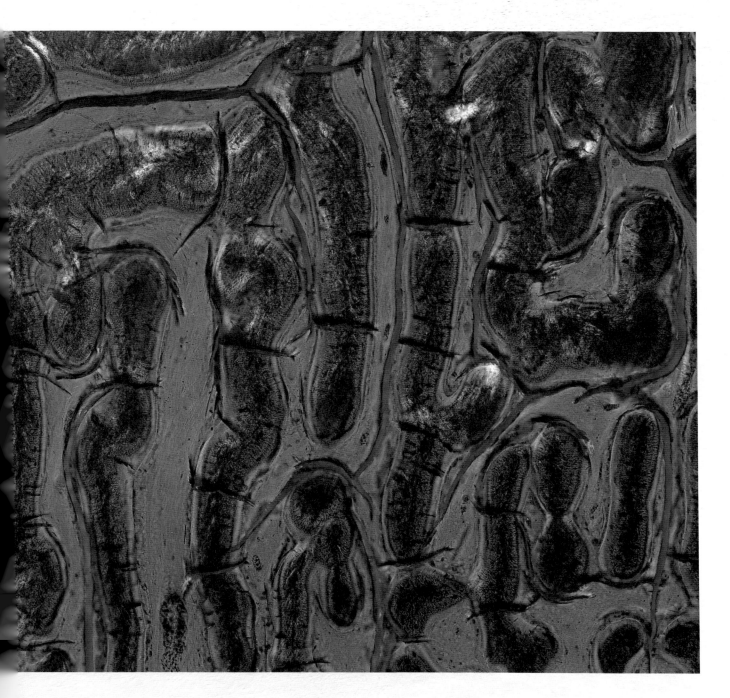

风骨 No.39

脱钙骨组织切片，X200，明视野，2016

Backbone No.39

Trabecular bone, Tissue section, X200, Light field, 2016

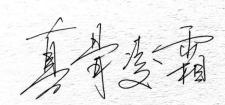

真骨凌霜

杨旭，46 岁，教授

Harsh frost tests real bone.

Yang Xu, 46, Professor

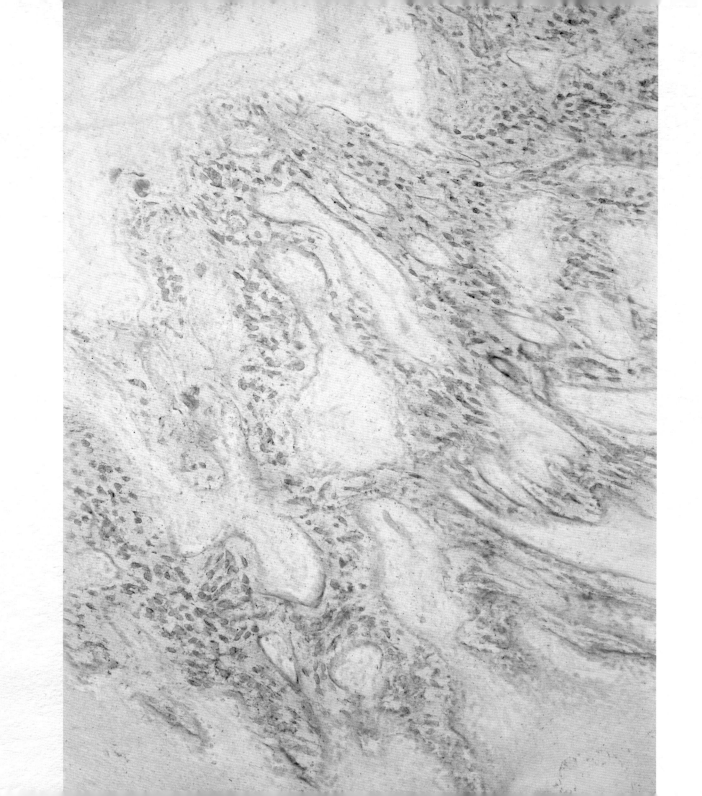

天书 No.151

未脱钙骨组织磨片，X40，明视野＋偏振光，2020

Heavenly script No.151

Trabecular bone, Ground section, X40, Light field + polarized light, 2020

字骨与诗魄

字骨与诗魄

董青，47 岁，教授

Bony character and poetic soul

Dong Qing, 47, Professor

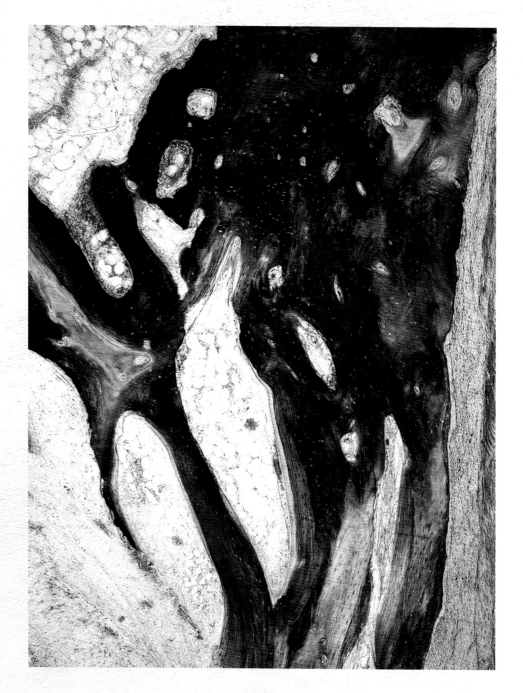

天书 No.38

脱钙骨组织切片，X40，明视野 + 偏振光，2013

Heavenly script No.38

Trabecular bone, Tissue section, X40, Light field + polarized light, 2013

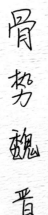

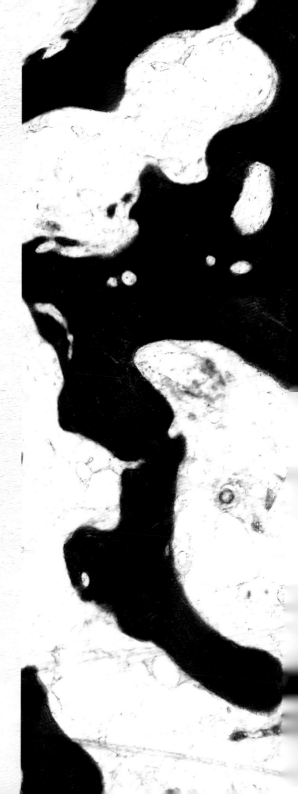

骨势魏晋

王琦芳，48 岁，酒店经理

Calligraphy style of Wei and Jin dynasties

Wang Qifang, 48, Hotel manager

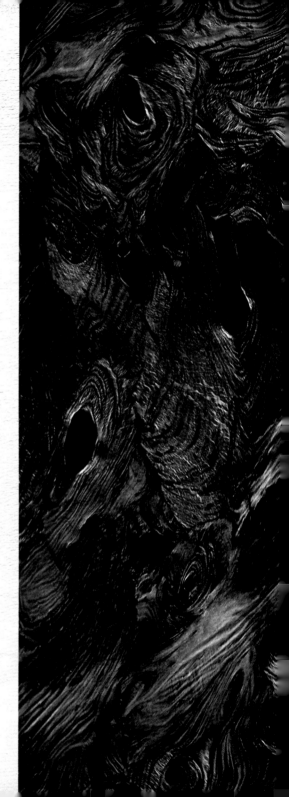

凝固的时间 No.6

脱钙骨组织切片，X40，偏振光，2017

Frozen time No.6

Cortical bone, Tissue section, X40, Polarized light, 2017

树没有前途，才在躯干上留下年轮。

黄锡荣，49 岁，金融职员

As there is no way ahead, trees leave the annual rings in their trunks.

Huang Xirong, 49, Financial staff

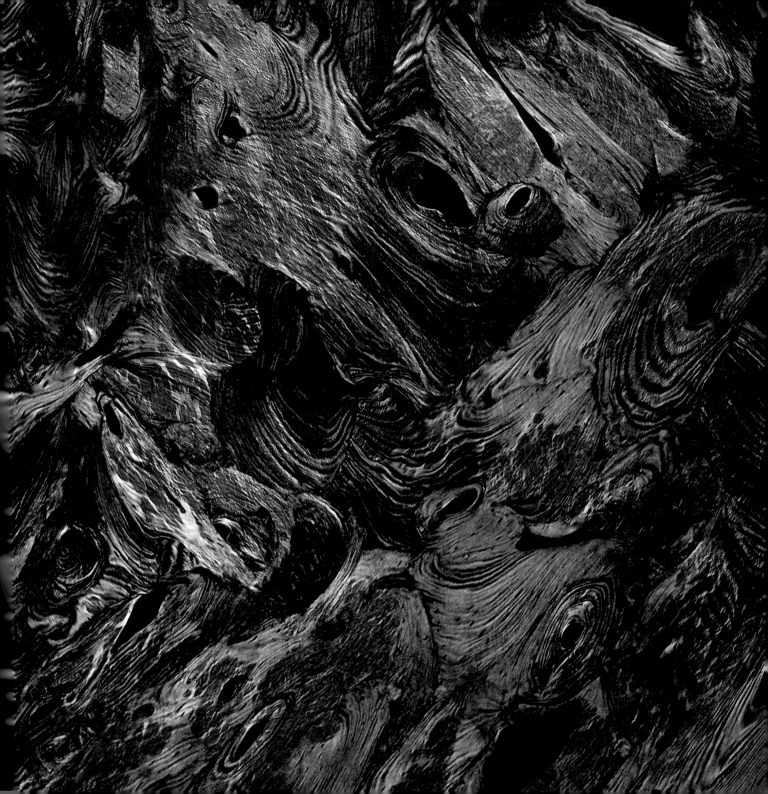

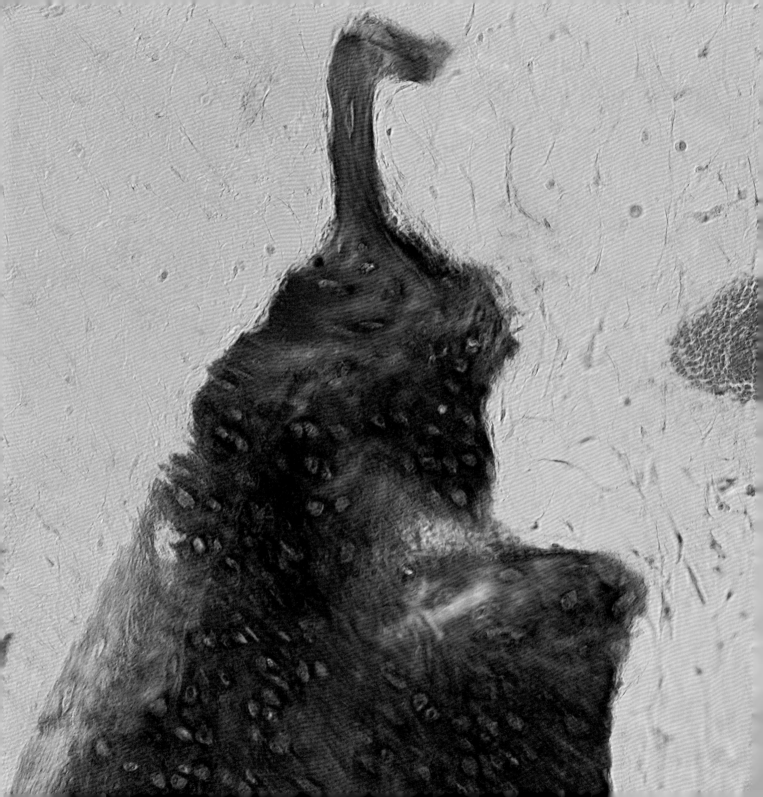

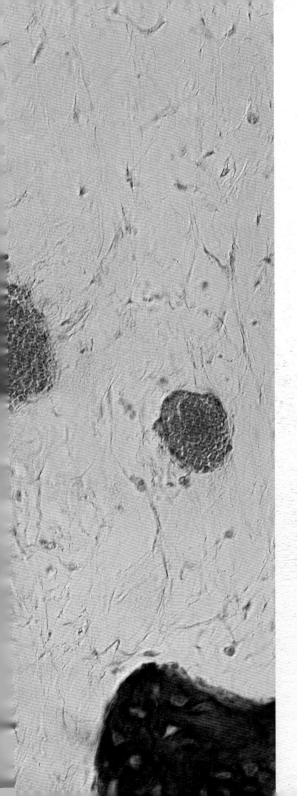

天书 No.86

未脱钙骨组织磨片，X100，明视野＋偏振光，2018

Heavenly script No.86

Trabecular bone, Ground section, X100, Light field + polarized light, 2018

生当作人杰，死亦为鬼雄。

李继红，50 岁，企业经理

Alive, be man of men; dead, be soul of souls.

Li Jihong, 50, Business manager

天书 No.157

未脱钙骨组织磨片，X40，明视野＋偏振光，2020

Heavenly script No.157

Trabecular bone, Ground section, X40, Light field
+ polarized light, 2020

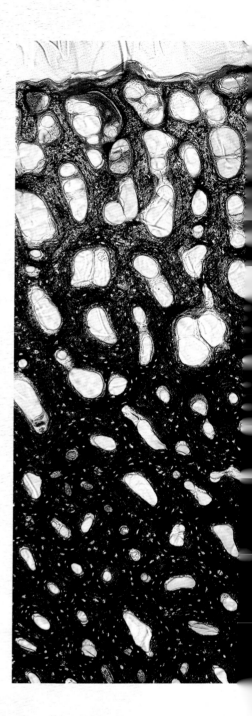

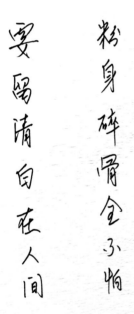

粉身碎骨全不怕，要留清白在人间。

胡小莉，51 岁，金融职员

Even if I have to be smashed to pieces,
I'll keep a clean slate in the world.

Hu Xiaoli, 51, Financial staff

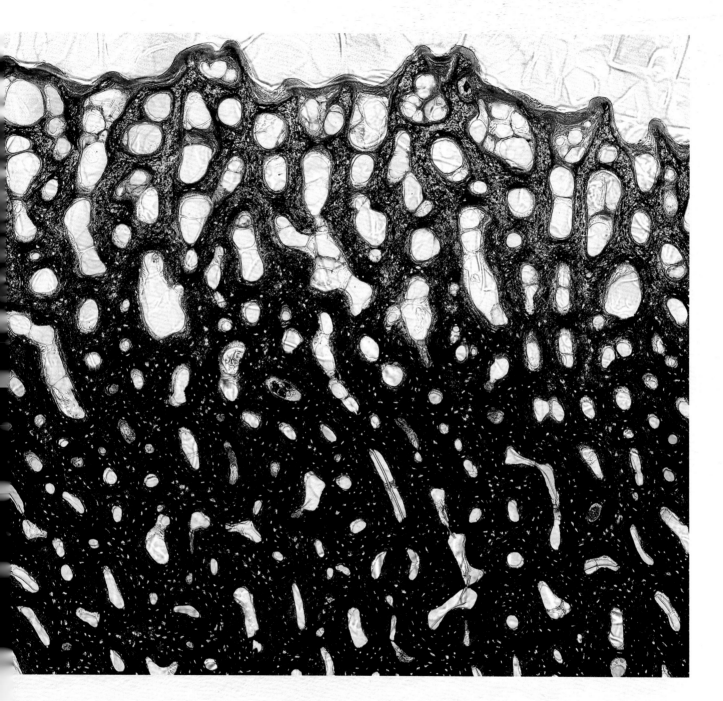

天书 No.129

未脱钙骨组织磨片，X200, 偏振光，2019

Heavenly script No.129

Cortical bone, Ground section, X200, Polarized light, 2019

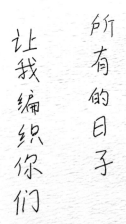

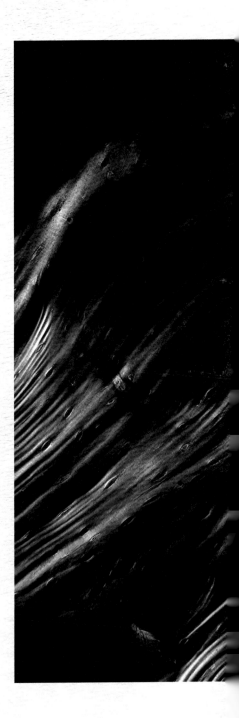

所有的日子，让我编织你们

俞强，52 岁，工程师

Come, the days ahead, let me weave you.

Yu Qiang, 52, Engineer

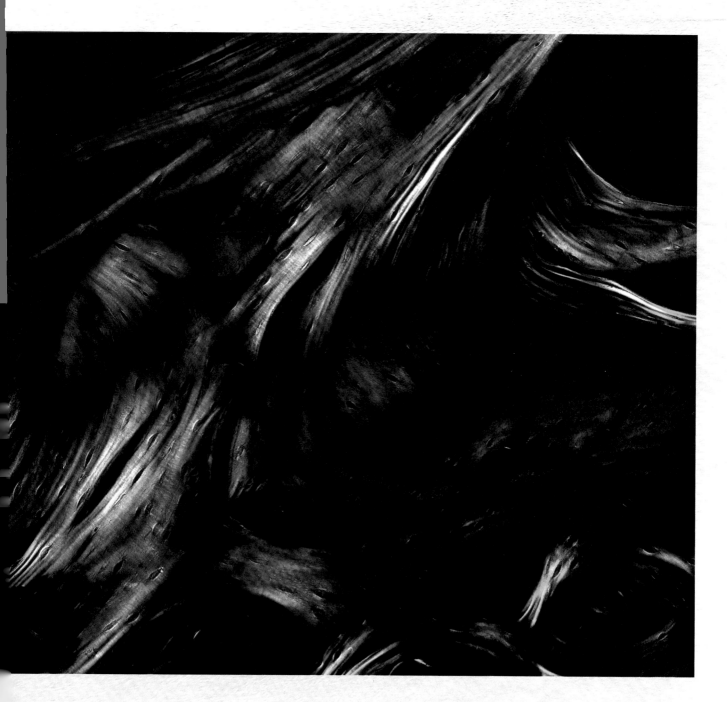

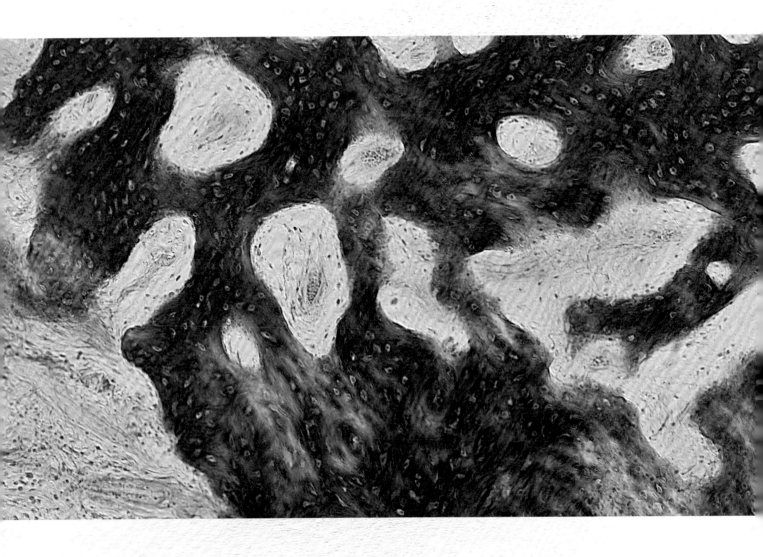

风骨 No.51

脱钙骨组织切片，X100，明视野 + 偏振光，2017

Backbone No.51

Trabecular bone, Tissue section, X100, Light field + polarized light, 2017

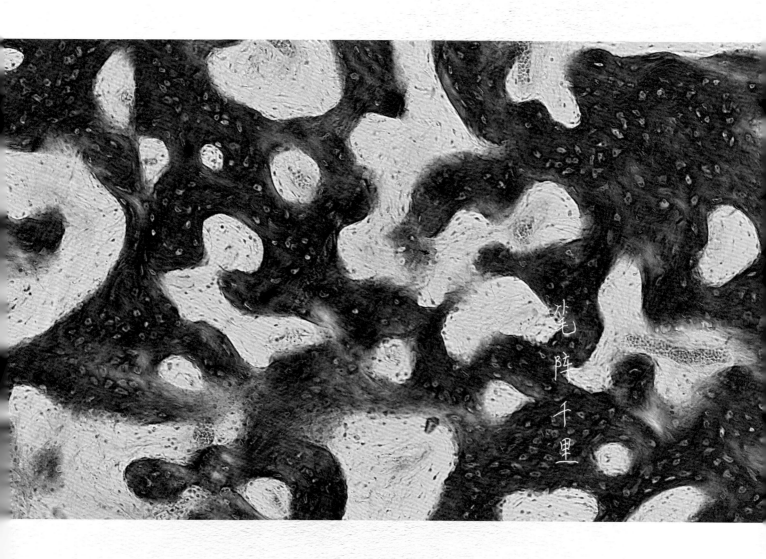

笔阵千里

笔阵千里

张春英，53 岁，工程师

The pen writing covers thousands of miles.

Zhang Chunying, 53, Engineer

风骨 No.53

脱钙骨组织切片，X100，偏振光，2017

Backbone No.53

Trabecular bone, Tissue section, X100, Polarized light, 2017

挥毫

李红叶，54 岁，主任医师

Wielding the writing brush

Li Hongye, 54, Head doctor

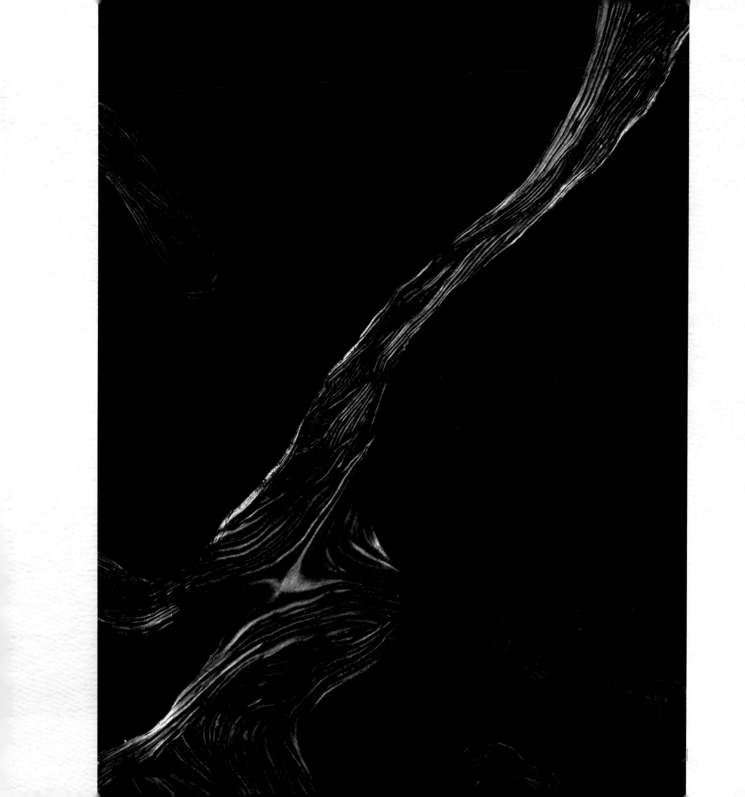

风骨 No.15

未脱钙骨组织磨片，X200, 偏振光，2013

Backbone No.15

Cortical bone, Ground section, X200, Polarized light, 2013

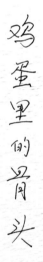

鸡蛋里的骨头

黄慧萍，55 岁，护士长

A bone in an egg

Huang Huiping, 55, Head nurse

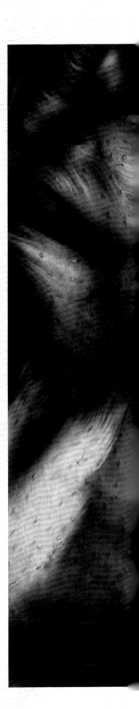

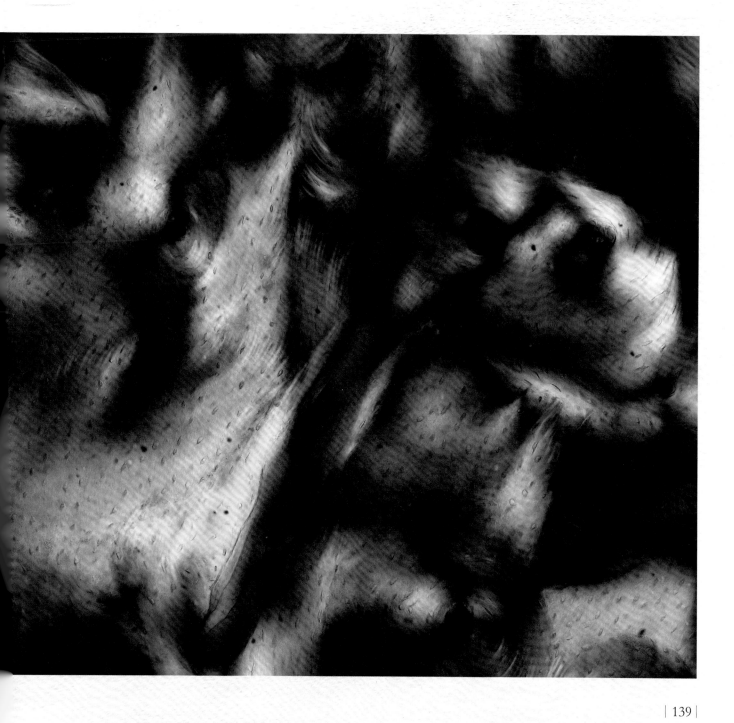

天书 No.2

脱钙骨组织切片，X200，明视野，2011

Heavenly script No.2

Trabecular bone, Tissue section, X200, Light field, 2011

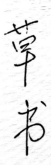

草书

董利民，56 岁，教授

Cursive script

Dong Limin, 56, Professor

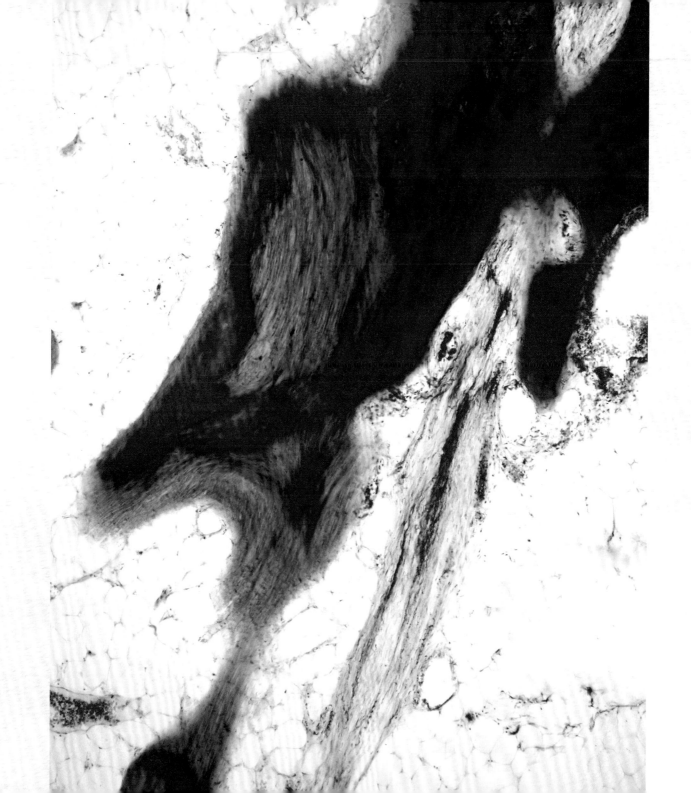

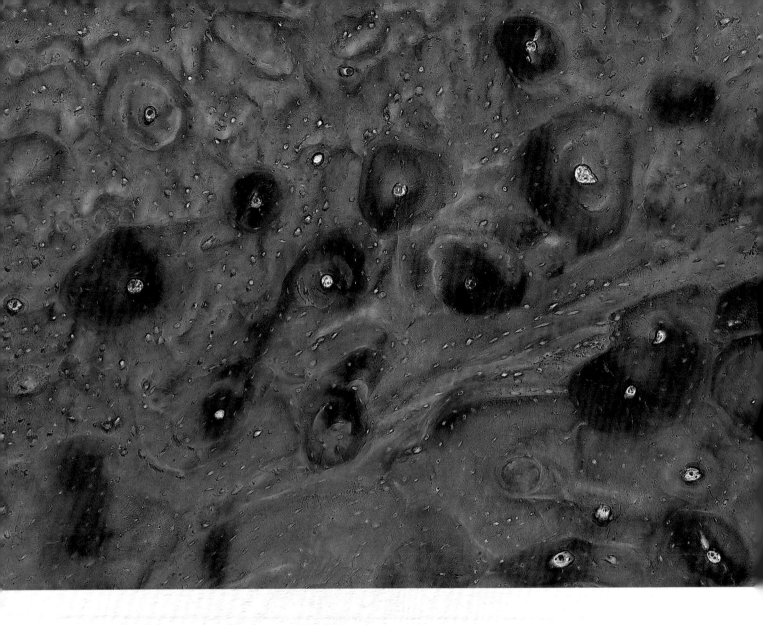

天书 No.170

未脱钙骨组织磨片，X40，明视野 + 偏振光，2021

Heavenly script No.170

Cortical bone, Ground section, X40, Light field + polarized light, 2021

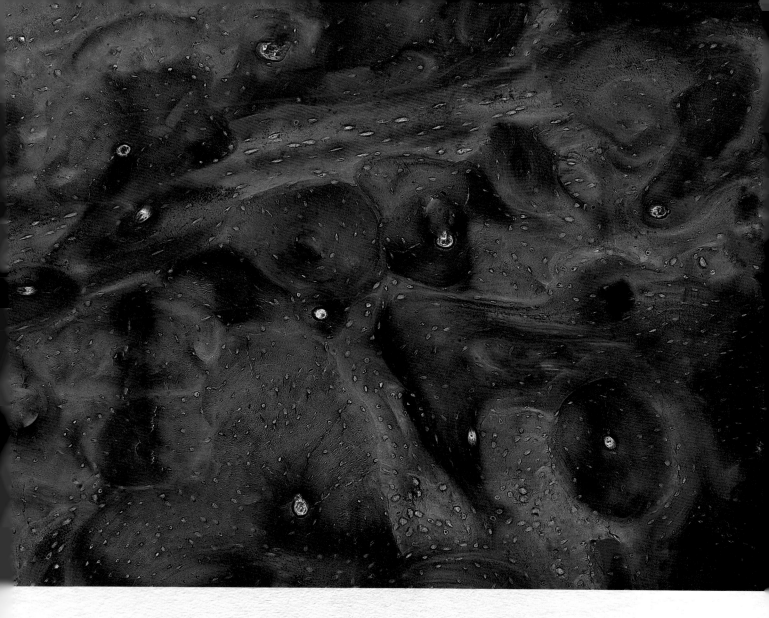

秀骨如碧

陈太辉，57 岁，公务员

Elegant bone as delicate as jade

Chen Taihui, 57, Civil servant

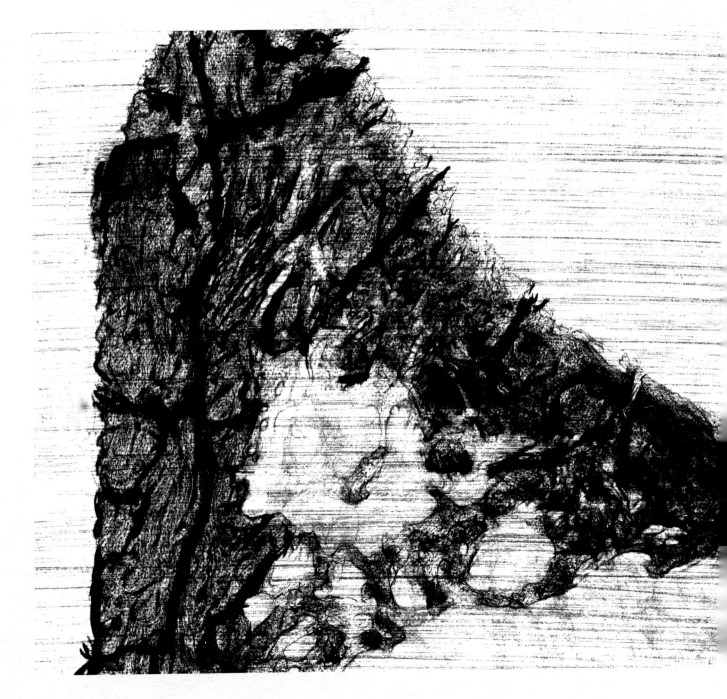

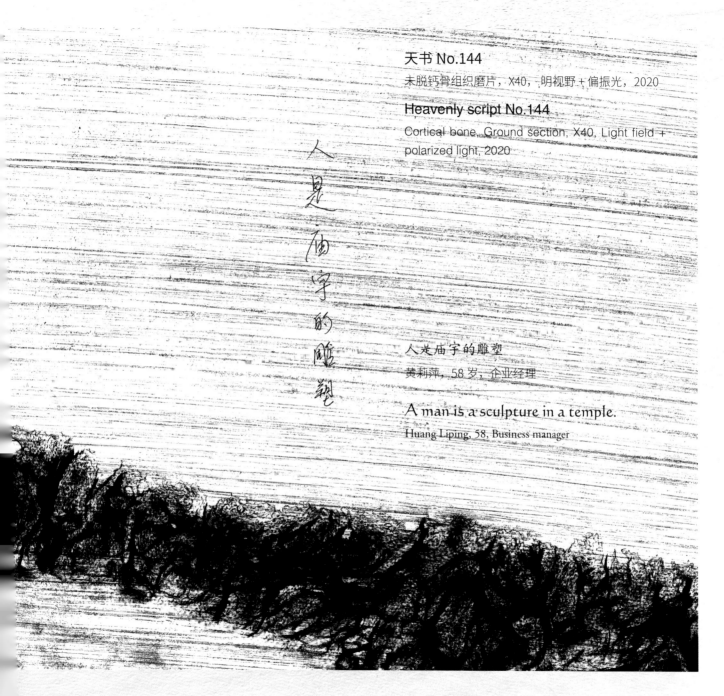

天书 No.144
未脱钙骨组织磨片，X40，明视野＋偏振光，2020

Heavenly script No.144
Cortical bone, Ground section, X40, Light field +
polarized light, 2020

人是庙宇的雕塑
黄莉萍，58 岁，企业经理

A man is a sculpture in a temple.
Huang Liping, 58, Business manager

植体的梦想 No.2

未脱钙骨组织和种植体磨片，X200，明视野 + 偏振光，2019

Dream of implant No.2

Implant with surrounding bone, Ground section, X200, Light
field + polarized light, 2019

玉骨冰姿

刘燕，59 岁，公司经理

Jade-like bone as graceful as ice

Liu Yan, 59, Company manager

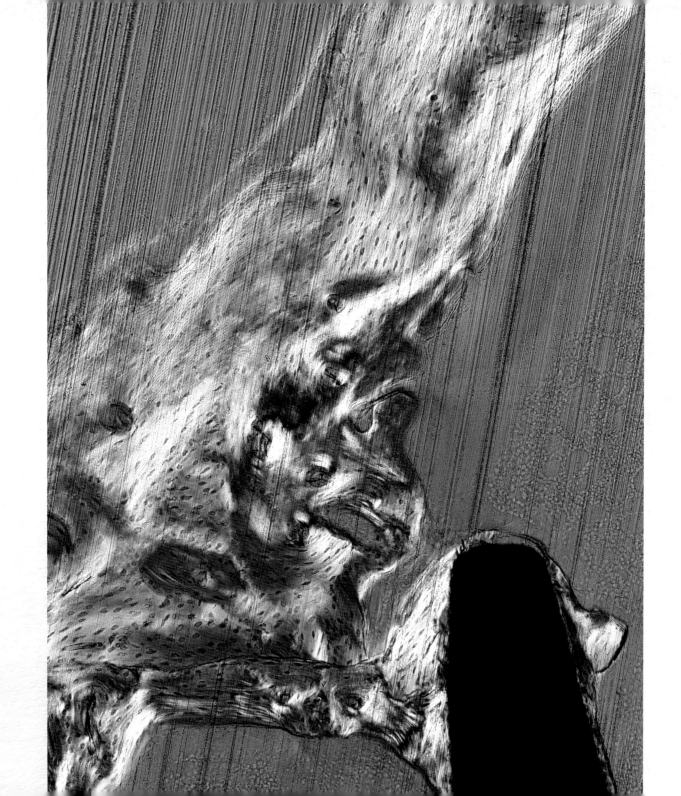

青花 No.2

未脱钙骨组织磨片，X100，偏振光，2013

Blue and white porcelain No.2

Trabecular bone, Ground section, X100, Polarized light, 2013

身体是灵魂作画的殿堂

李铁军，60 岁，教授

The human body is the temple where the soul paints.

Li Tiejun, 60, Professor

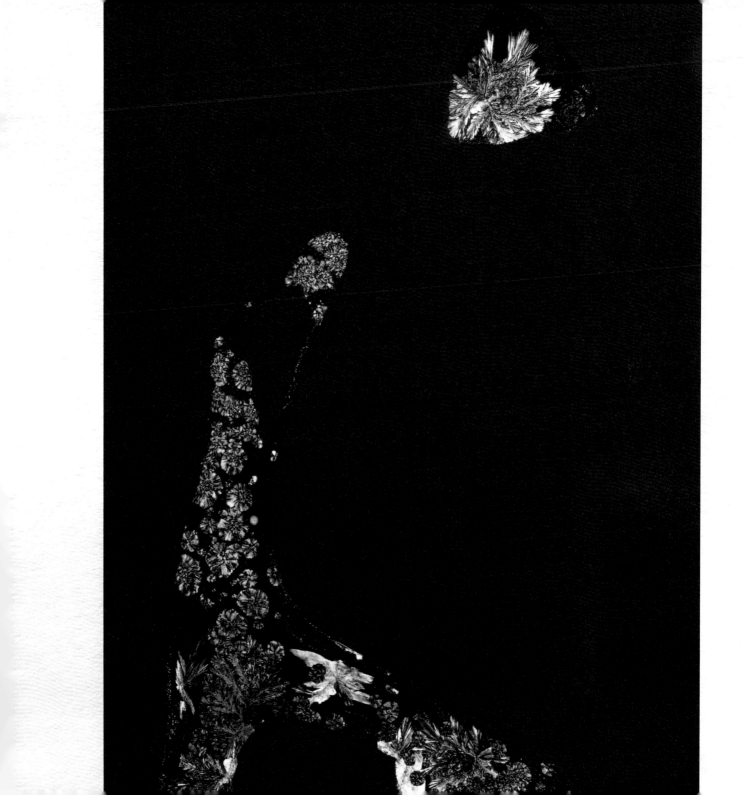

天书 No.134

未脱钙骨组织磨片，X100，明视野＋偏振光，2020

Heavenly script No.134

Trabecular bone, Ground section, X100, Light field
+ polarized light, 2020

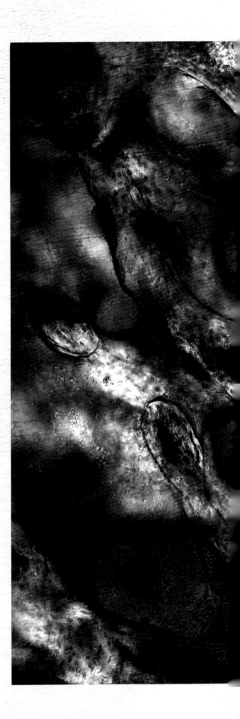

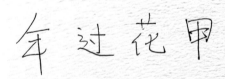

年过花甲

周桂兰，61 岁，教授

Well over sixty

Zhou Guilan, 61, Professor

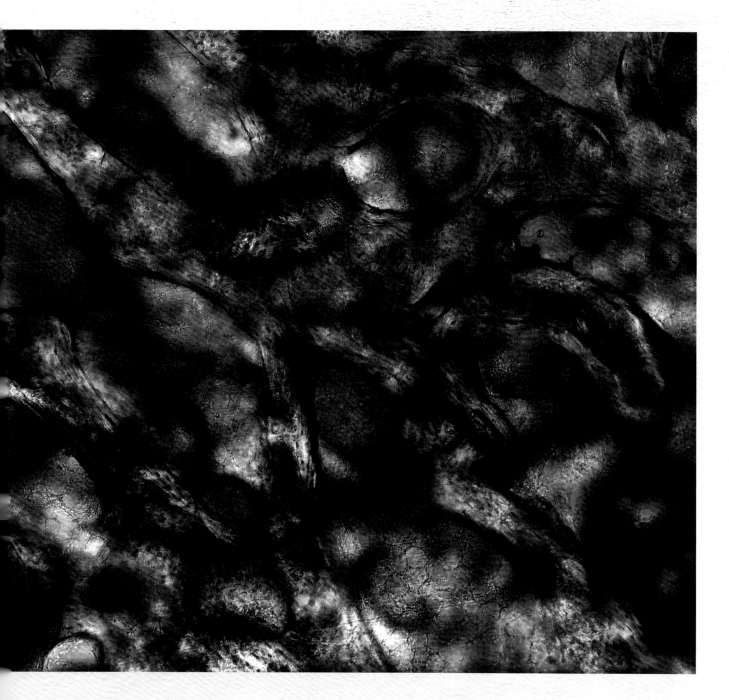

甲骨文 No.5

未脱钙骨组织磨片，X40，明视野 + 偏振光，2020

Oracle No.5

Trabecular bone, Ground section, X40, Light field + polarized light, 2020

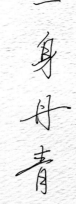

一身丹青

李翠英，62 岁，教授

Dressed in red and blue

Li Cuiying, 62, Professor

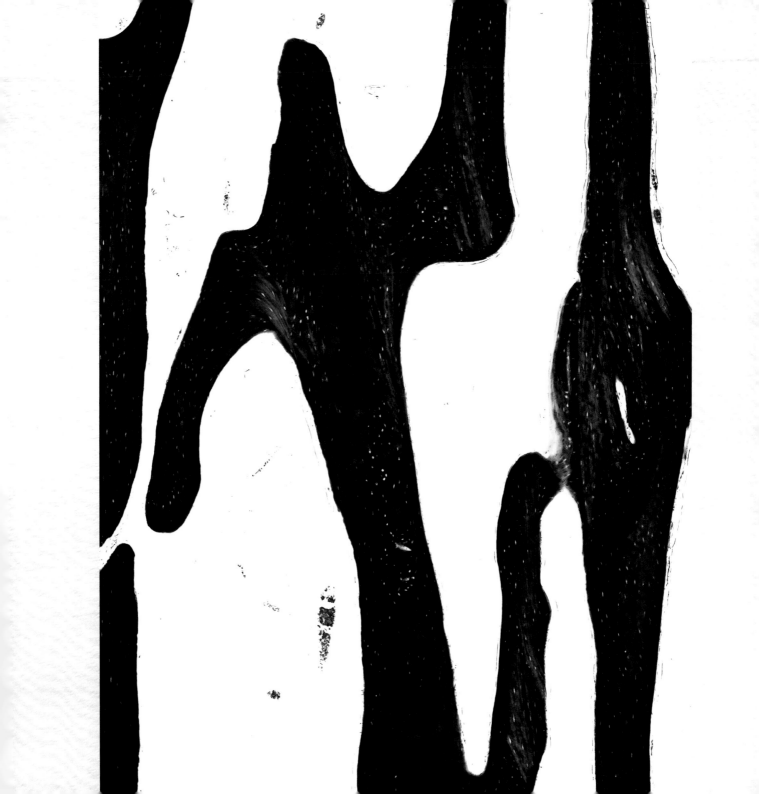

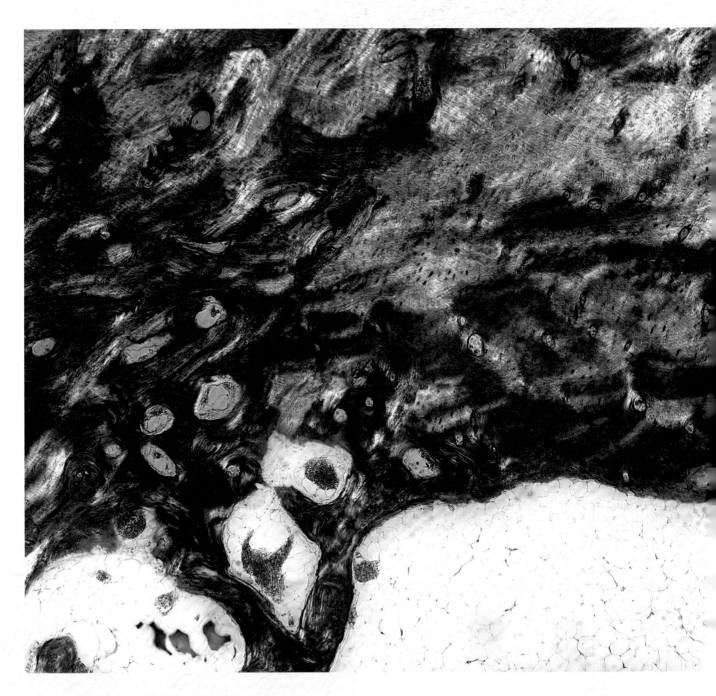

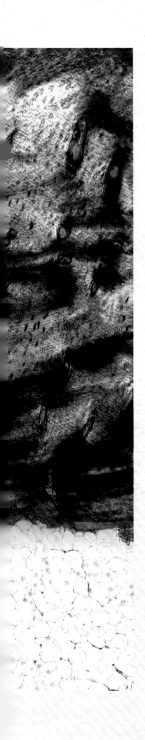

蓝色的树

未脱钙骨组织磨片，X40，明视野 + 偏振光，2020

Blue tree

Trabecular bone, Ground section, X40, Light field + polarized light, 2020

风骨可鉴

刘宝生，63 岁

Bone's proud integrity

Liu Baosheng, 63

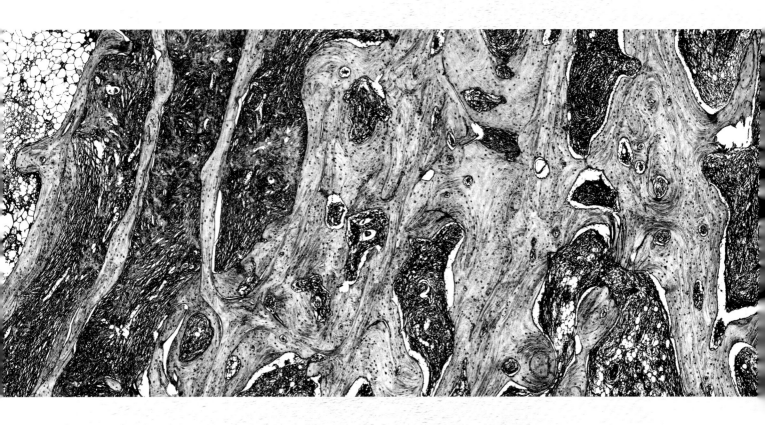

天书 No.138

未脱钙骨组织磨片，X40，明视野 + 偏振光，2020

Heavenly script No.138

Trabecular bone, Ground section, X40, Light field + polarized light, 2020

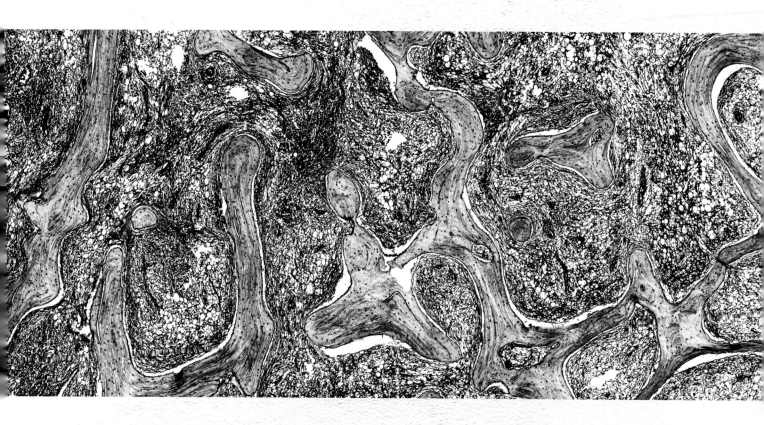

凡胎浊骨

杨立强，64 岁，企业经理

The body as heir to all mortal desires

Yang Liqiang, 64, Business manager

天书 No.61

脱钙骨组织切片，X40，偏振光，2014

Heavenly script No.61

Trabecular bone, Tissue section, X40, Polarized light, 2014

作别

韩凤云，65 岁，退休教师

Bid farewell

Han Fengyun, 65, Retired teacher

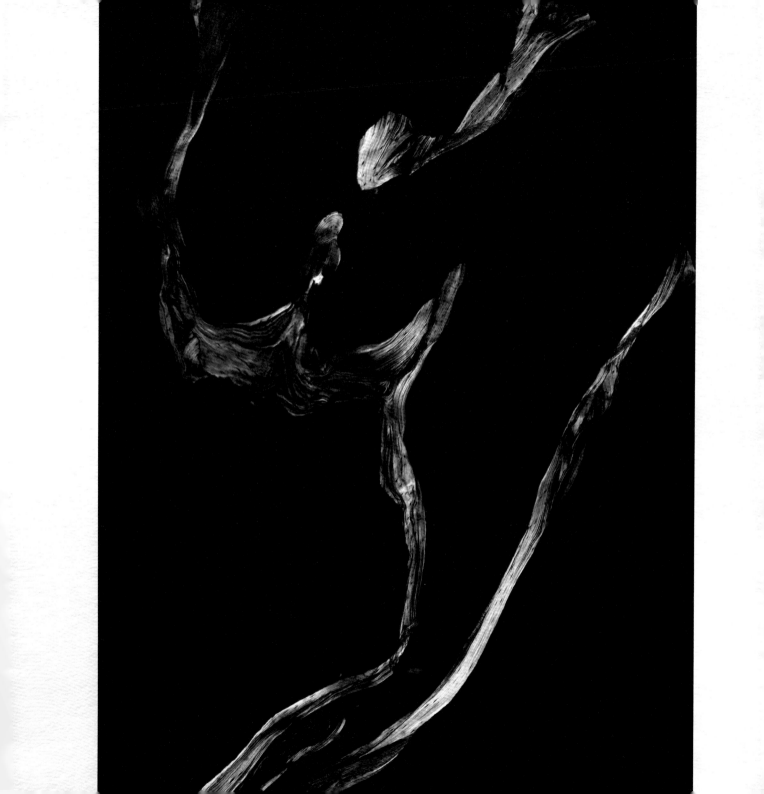

流星雨 No.4

未脱钙骨组织磨片，X100，偏振光，2020

Meteor shower No.4

Cortical bone tissues, Ground section, X100, Polarized light, 2020

天边的云彩

天边的云彩

汪照育，66 岁

Colorful clouds in the sky

Wang Zhaoyu, 66

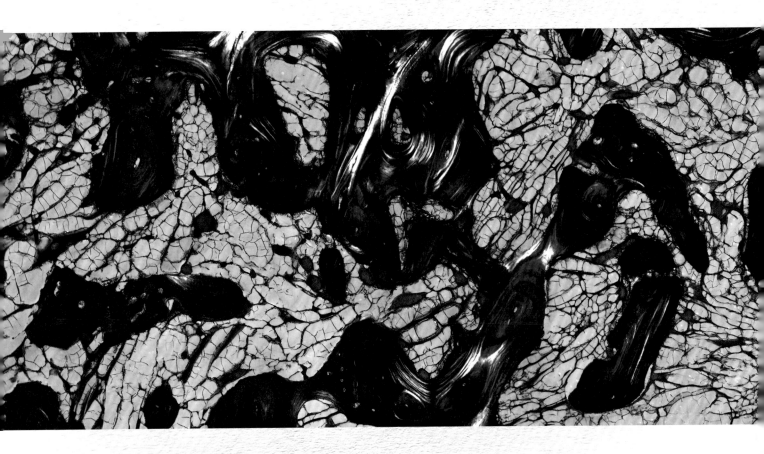

漆画

未脱钙骨组织磨片，X40，明视野 + 偏振光，2019

Lacquer painting

Trabecular bone, Ground section, X40, Light field + polarized light, 2019

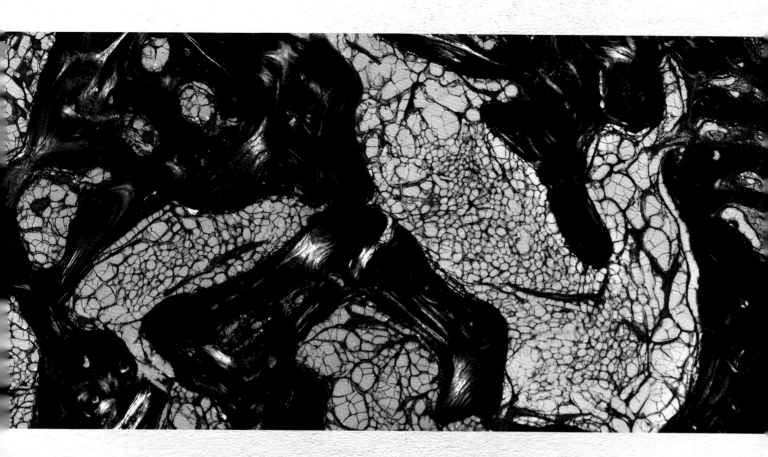

身体的壁画

身体的壁画
董化斌，67 岁

Mural of the body
Dong Huabin, 67

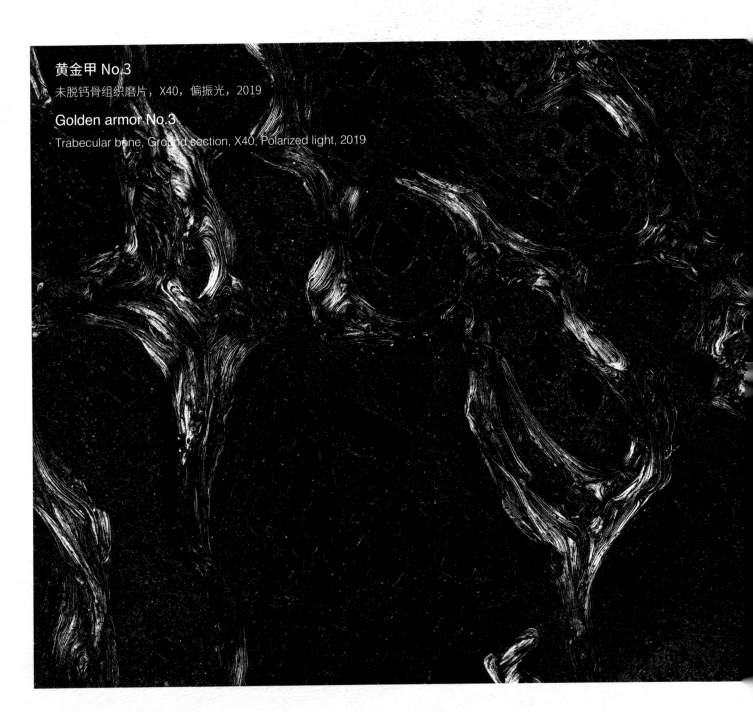

黄金甲 No.3

未脱钙骨组织磨片，X40，偏振光，2019

Golden armor No.3

Trabecular bone, Ground section, X40, Polarized light, 2019

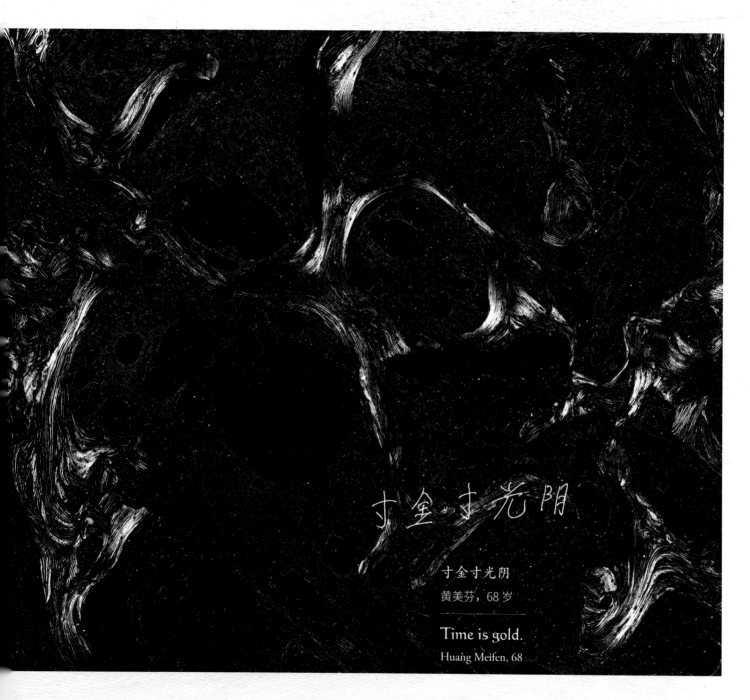

寸金寸光阴

寸金寸光阴
黄美芬，68 岁

Time is gold.
Huang Meifen, 68

天书 No.150

未脱钙骨组织磨片，X100，偏振光，2020

Heavenly script No.150

Cortical bone tissues, Ground section, X100, Polarized light, 2020

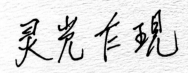

灵光乍现

朱国良，69 岁

Flash of halo

Zhu Guoliang, 69

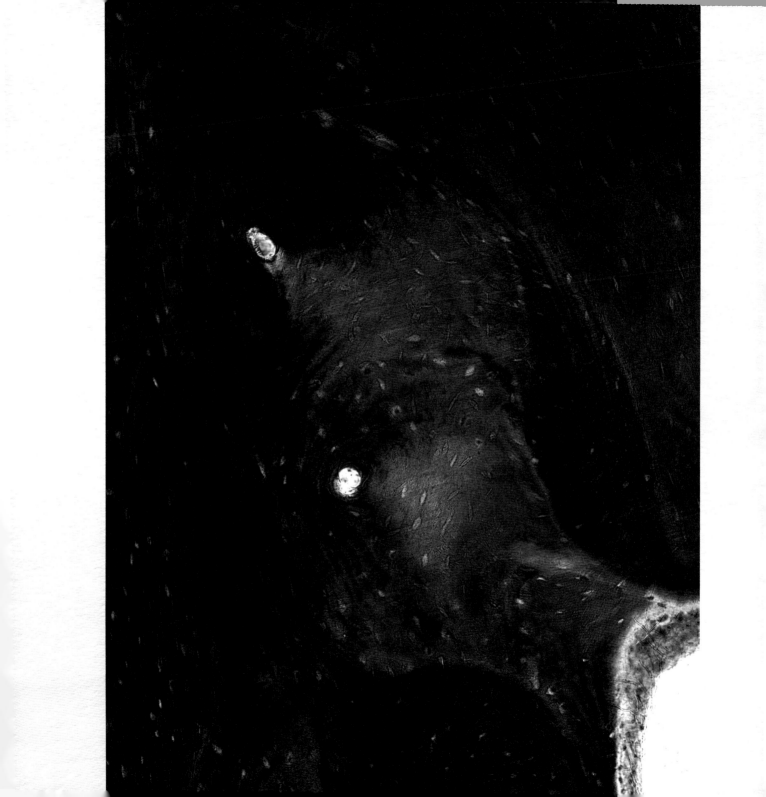

天书 No.79

脱钙骨组织切片，X100，偏振光，2017

Heavenly script No.79

Cortical bone, Tissue section, X100, Polarized light, 2017

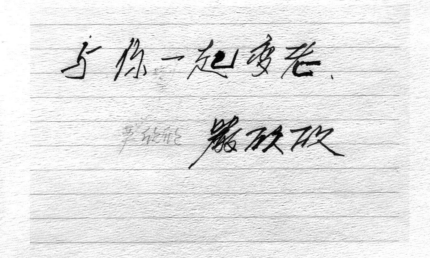

与你一起变老

严欣欣，70 岁

To grow old together with you

Yan Xinxin, 70

空山 No.2

未脱钙磨片，骨关节处的骨与覆盖表面的软骨以及

周围的封片胶，X12.5，明视野＋偏振光，2021

Empty mountain No.2

Bone and surface covered cartilage with sealing
gel, Ground section, X12.5, Light field + polarized
light, 2021

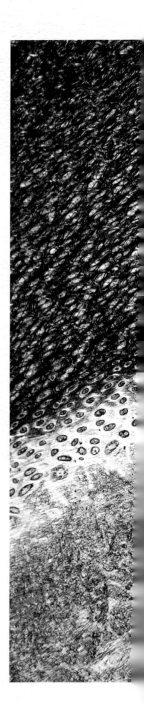

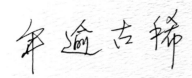

年逾古稀

胡德华，71 岁

In my seventies

Hu Dehua, 71

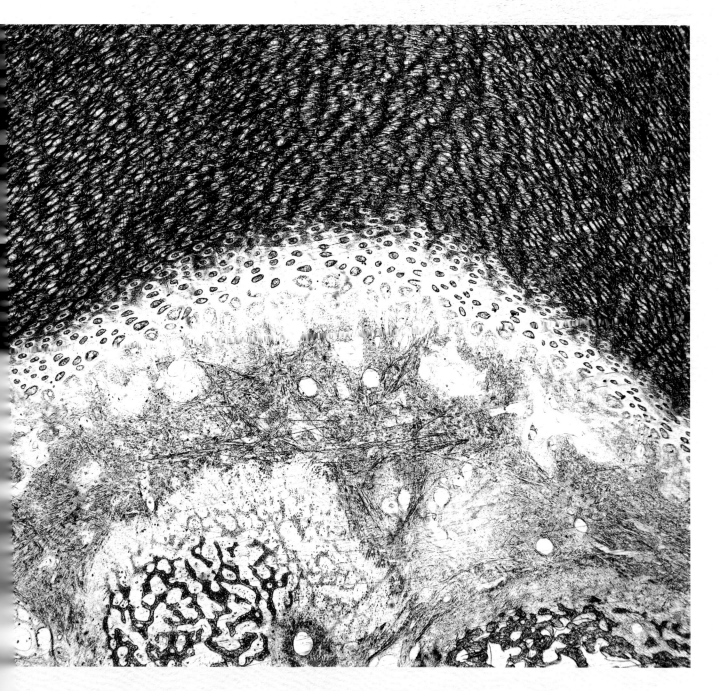

风骨 No.59

未脱钙骨组织磨片，X100，偏振光，2019

Backbone No.59

Trabecular bone, Ground section, X100,
Polarized light, 2019

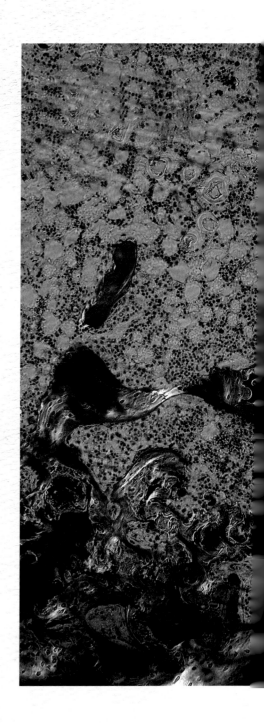

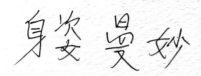

身姿曼妙
黄美英，72 岁

A graceful posture

Huang Meiying, 72

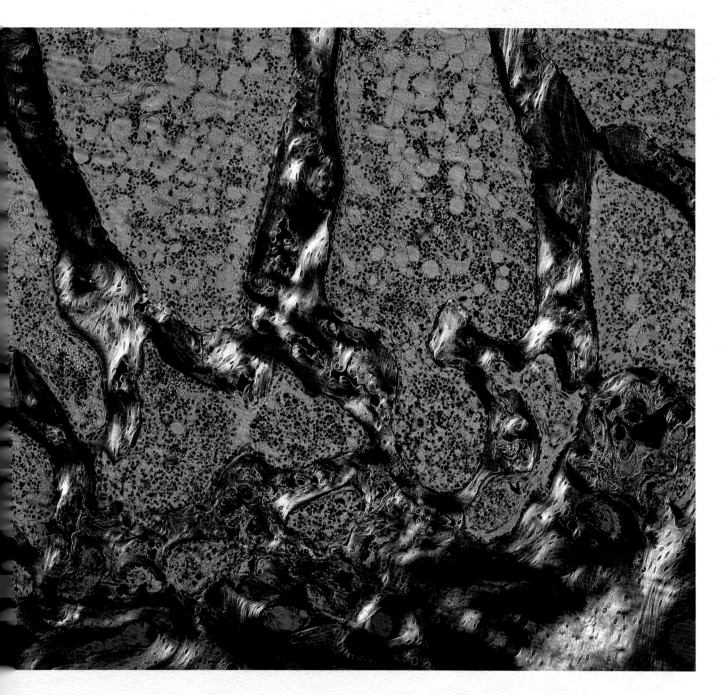

天书 No.63

未脱钙骨组织磨片，X100，偏振光，2015

Heavenly script No.63

Trabecular bone, Ground section, X100, Polarized light, 2015

鹤舞晨光

鹤舞晨光

郭家麟，73 岁

A crane dances in the morning light.

Guo Jialin, 73

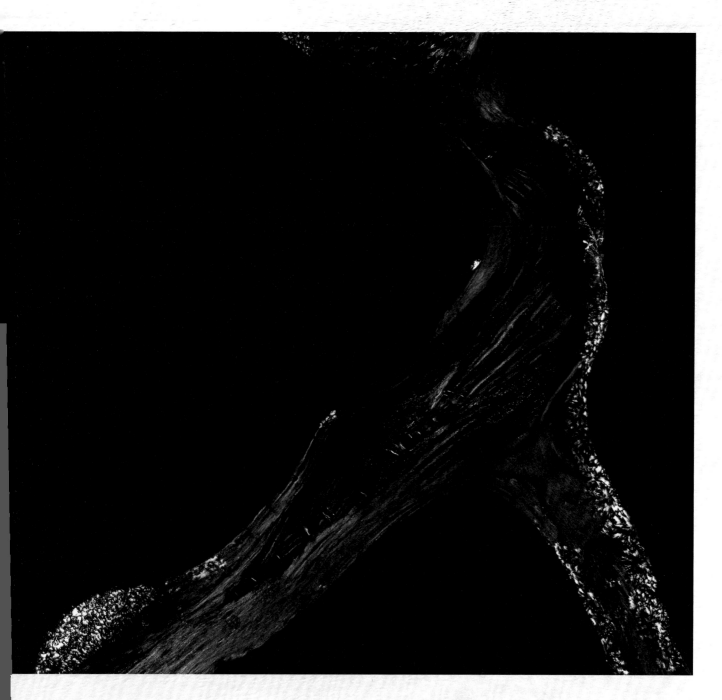

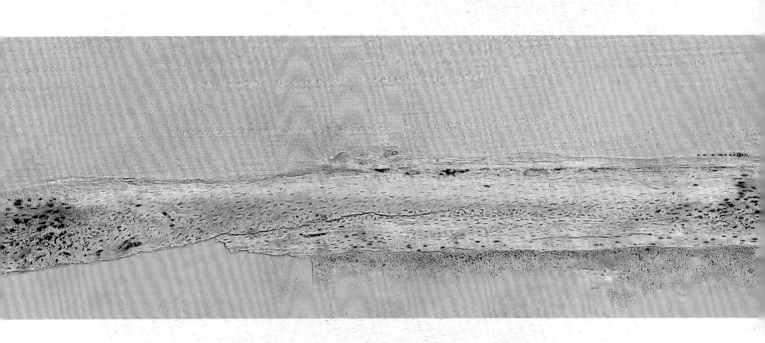

雪原

未脱钙骨组织与人工填料磨片，X100，明视野 + 偏振光，2019

Snowfield

Bone tissue with implanted materials, Ground section, X100, Light field + polarized light, 2019

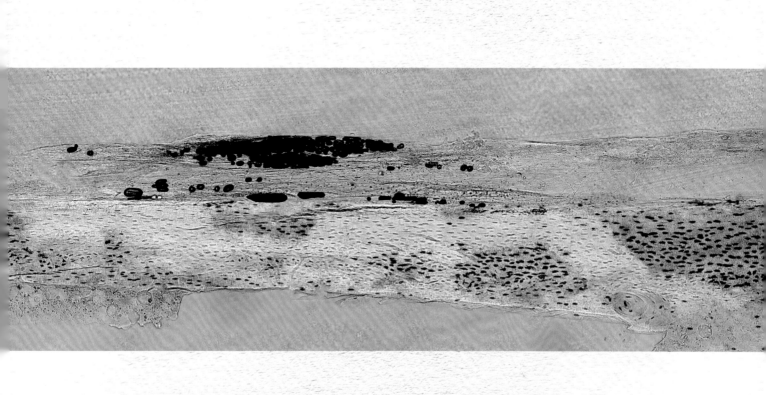

冰雪寒山

冰雪寒山
皇甫临沛，74 岁

Snow-covered mountains
Huangfu Linpei, 74

天书 No.143

未脱钙骨组织磨片，X100，偏振光，2020

Heavenly script No.143

Cortical bone, Ground section, X100, Polarized light, 2020

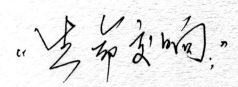

生命交响

袁玉贵，75 岁

Symphony of life

Yuan Yugui, 75

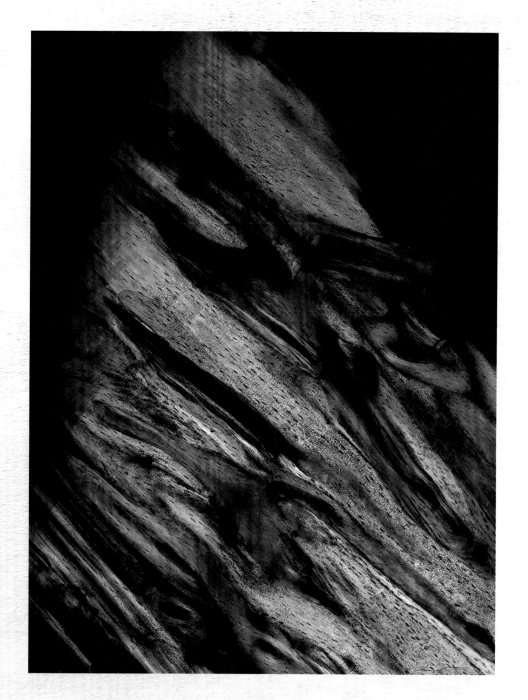

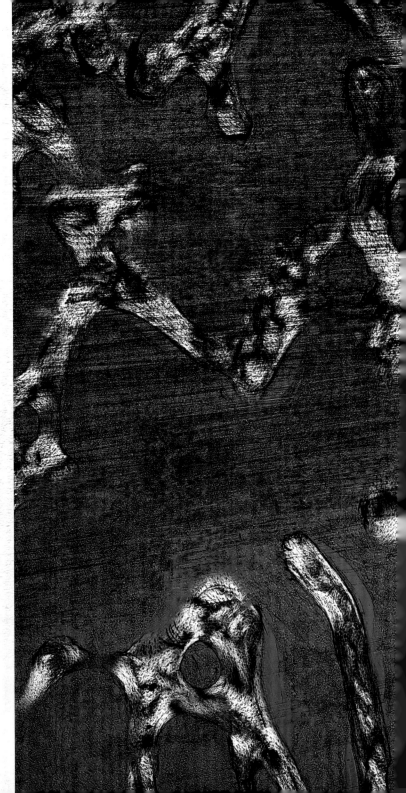

天书 No.196

未脱钙骨组织磨片，X40，偏振光，2021

Heavenly script No.196

Trabecular bone, Ground section, X40, Polarized light, 2021

硬 骨 头

硬骨头

李文燕，76 岁

Iron hard bone

Li Wenyan, 76

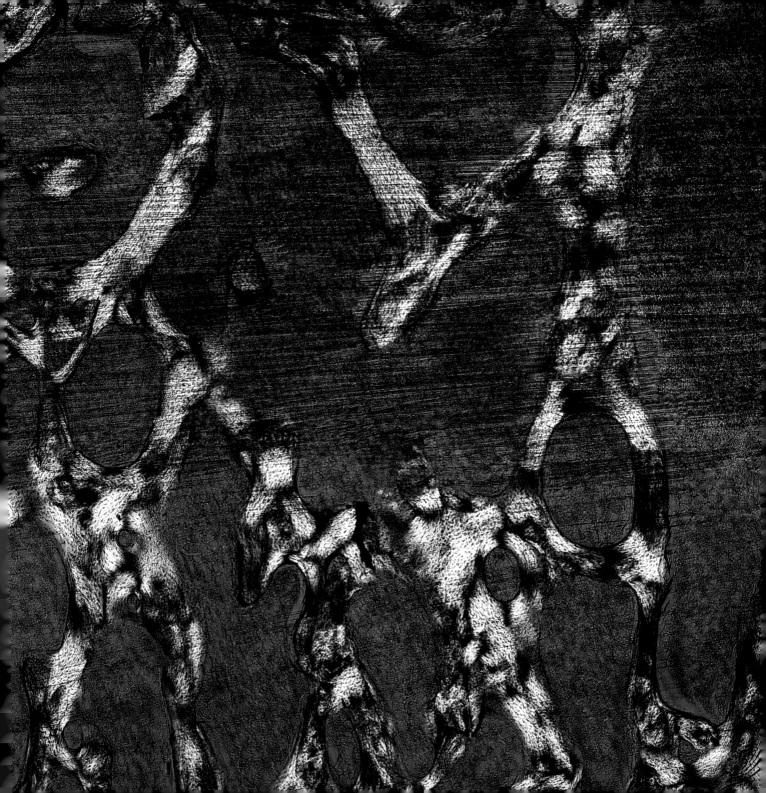

风骨 No.16

脱钙骨组织切片，X100，偏振光，2013

Backbone No.16

Trabecular bone, Tissue section, X100, Polarized light, 2013

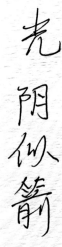

光 阴 似 箭

崔玉娥，77 岁

How time flies.

Cui Yu'e, 77

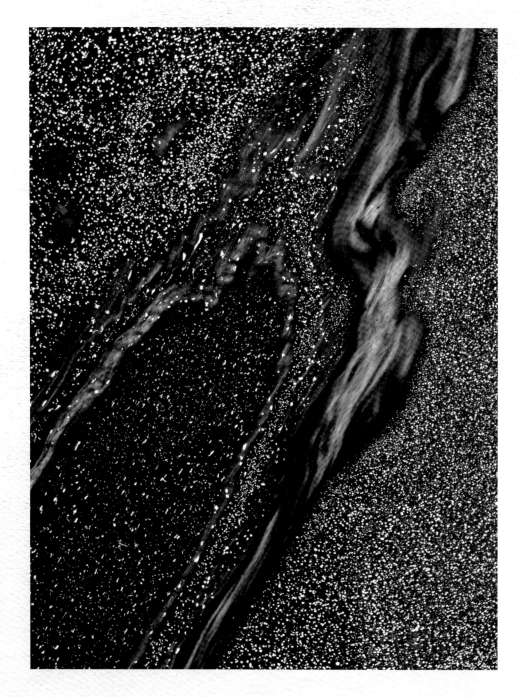

天书 No.28

未脱钙骨组织磨片，X40， 偏振光，2013

Heavenly script No.28

Trabecular bone, Ground section, X40, Polarized light, 2013

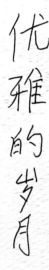

优雅的岁月

吕淑柏，78 岁

The years of grace

Lv Shubo, 78

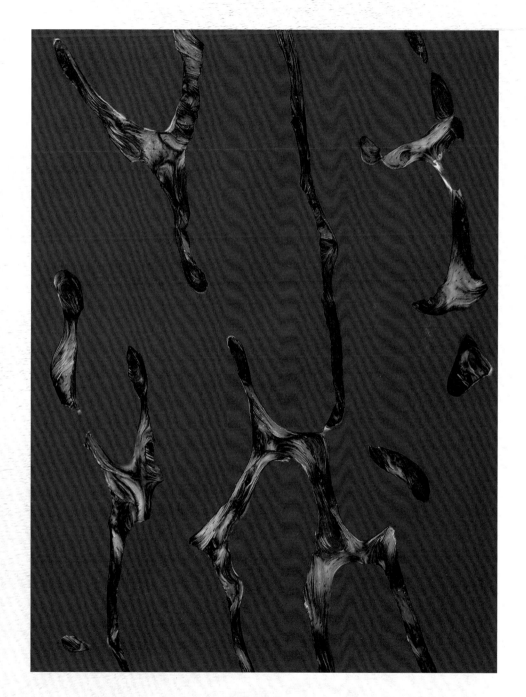

风骨 No.17

未脱钙骨组织磨片，X200，偏振光，2013

Backbone No.17

Trabecular bone, Ground section, X200, Polarized light, 2013

过去的不都是往事

张乐山，79 岁

History is not always recollections of the past.

Zhang Leshan, 79

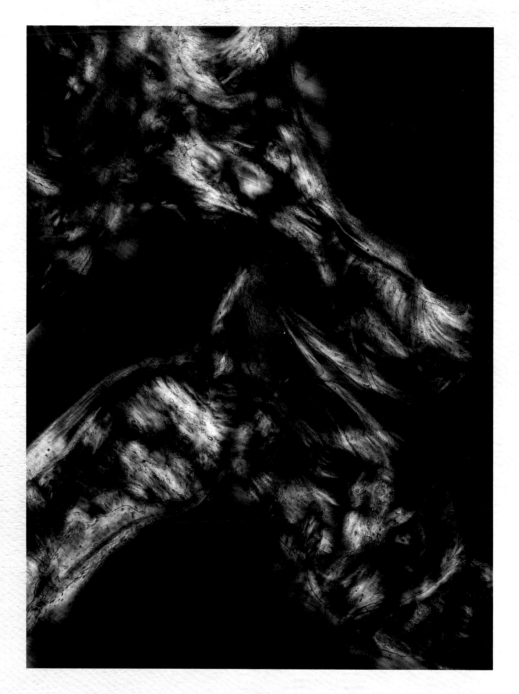

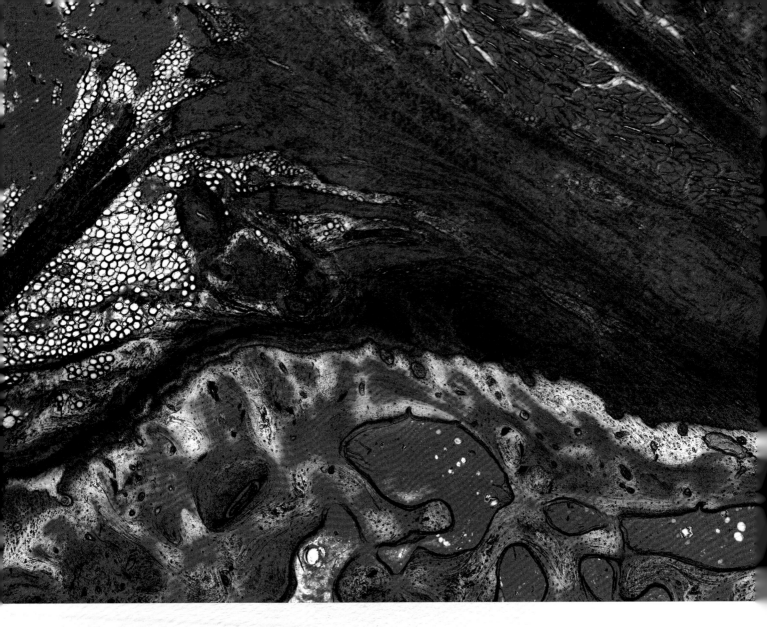

秋色漫山 No.2

未脱钙骨及肌肉组织磨片，X40，明视野＋偏振光，2019

Autumn-tinged mountains No.2

Bone and muscles, Ground section, X 40, Light field + polarized light, 2019

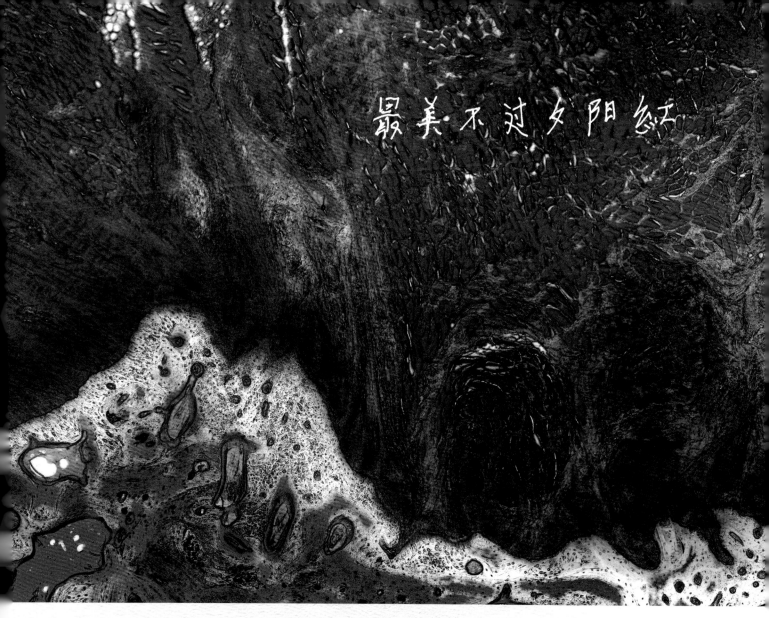

最美不过夕阳红

顾如玉，80岁

Nothing is more beautiful than the splendor of sunset.

Gu Ruyu, 80

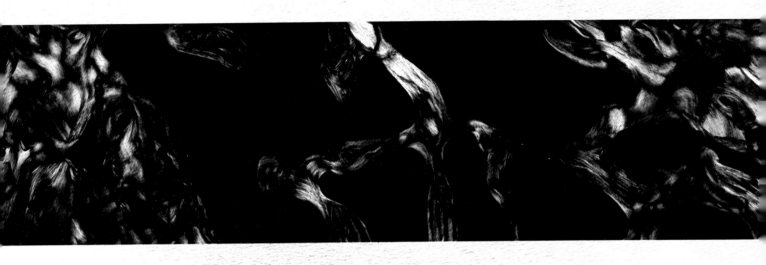

风骨 No.38

脱钙骨组织切片，X40，偏振光，2016

Backbone No.38

Trabecular bone, Tissue section, X40, Polarized light, 2016

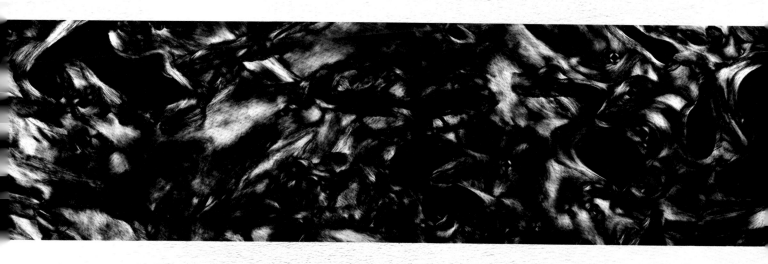

此心安处是吾乡

此心安处是吾乡

叶秀荣，81 岁

Home is where heart finds
freedom from worries.

Ye Xiurong, 81

龙骨

脱钙骨组织切片，X200，明视野 + 偏振光，2011

Bone of dragon

Trabecular bone, Tissue section, X200, Light field + polarized light, 2011

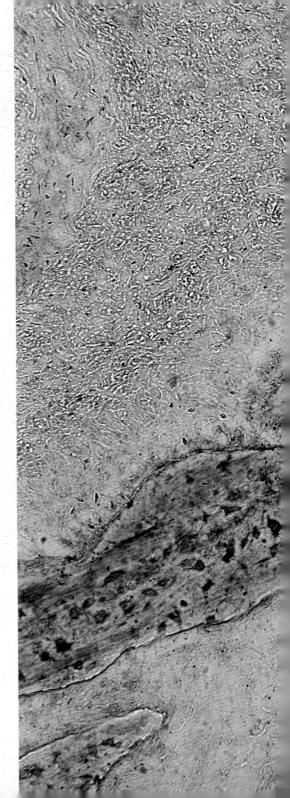

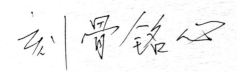

刻骨铭心

杨增庆，82 岁

Imprinted on the bones and inscribed on the memory

Yang Zengqing, 82

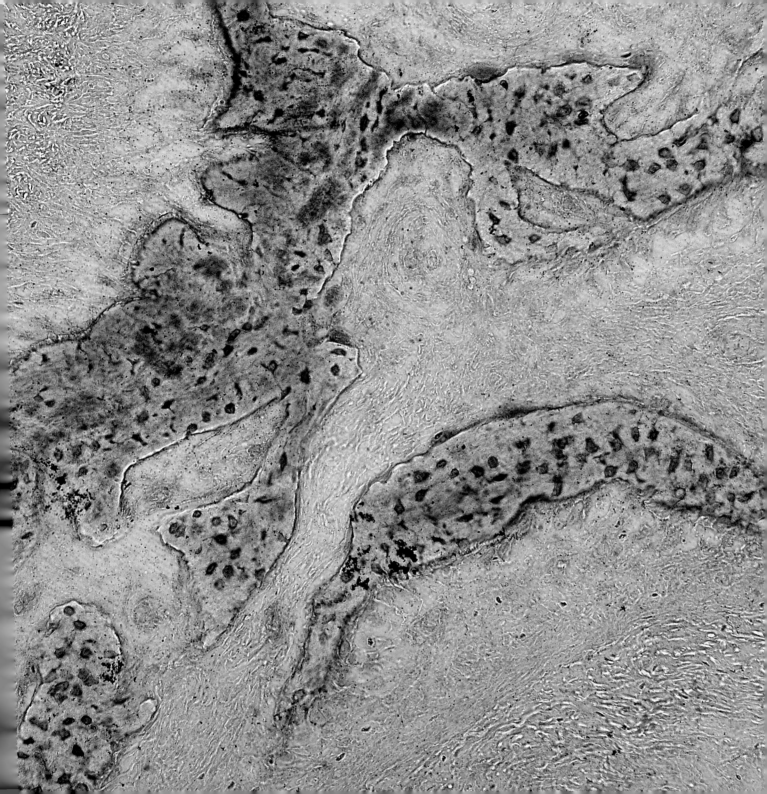

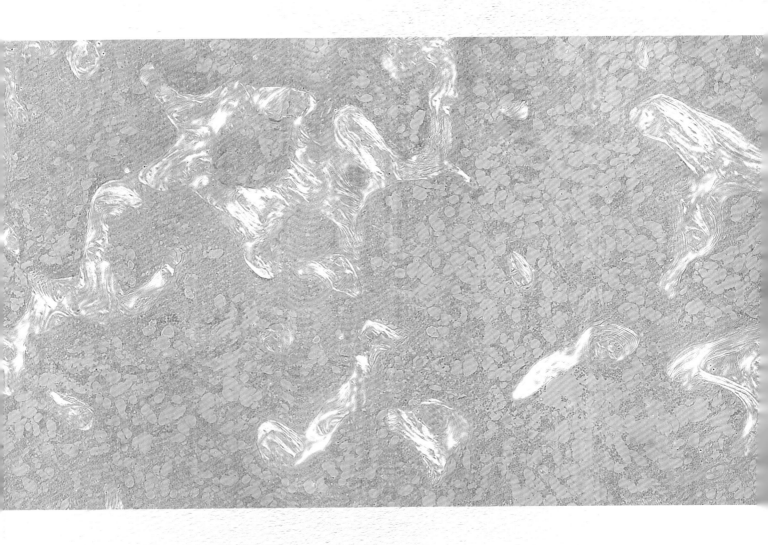

天书 No.189

未脱钙骨组织磨片，X100，偏振光，2021

Heavenly script No.189

Trabecular bone, Ground section, X100, Polarized light, 2021

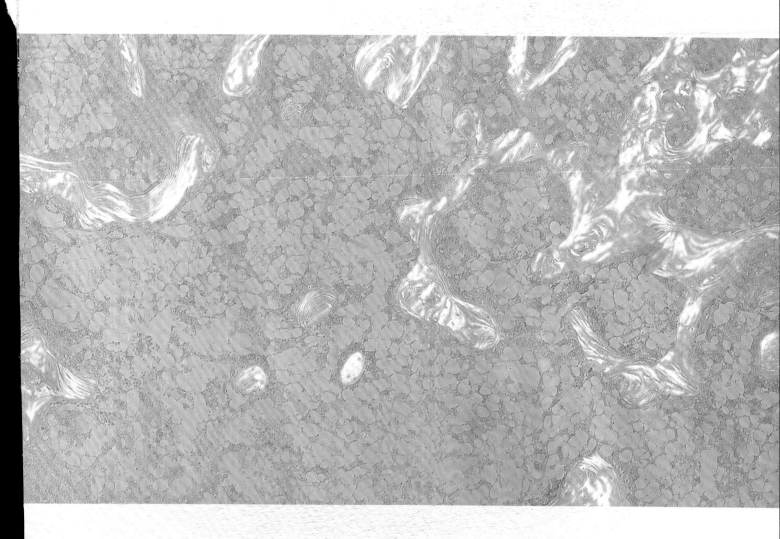

雪胎梅骨

雪胎梅骨
李仁杰，83 岁

Life wrapped in snow protected
by plum's bone
Li Renjie, 83

大山

未脱钙骨及周围软组织磨片，X40，明视野 + 偏振光，2020

The mountain

Cortical bone and soft tissues, Ground section, X40, Light field + polarized light, 2020

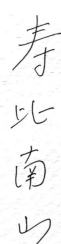

寿比南山

黄永全，84 岁

Live as long as the Southern Mountain

Huang Yongquan, 84

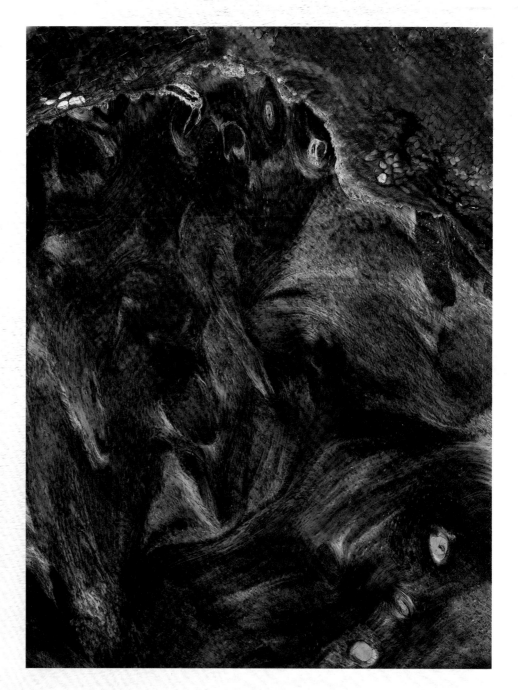

红丝带

脱钙骨组织切片，X100，偏振光，2013

Red ribbon

Trabecular bone, Tissue section, X100, Polarized light, 2013

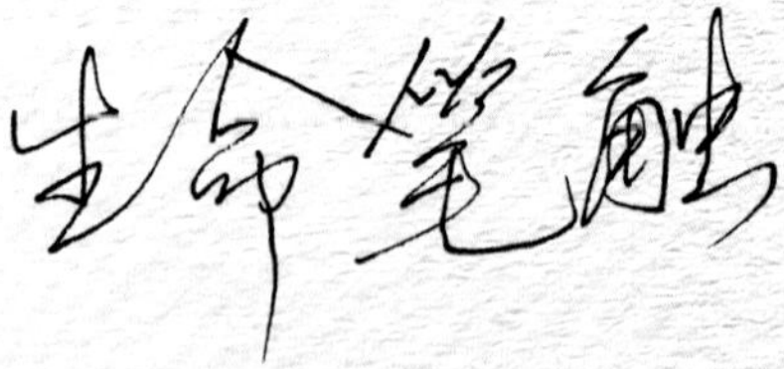

生命笔触

高齐瑜，85岁

The brush strokes of life

Gao Qiyu, 85

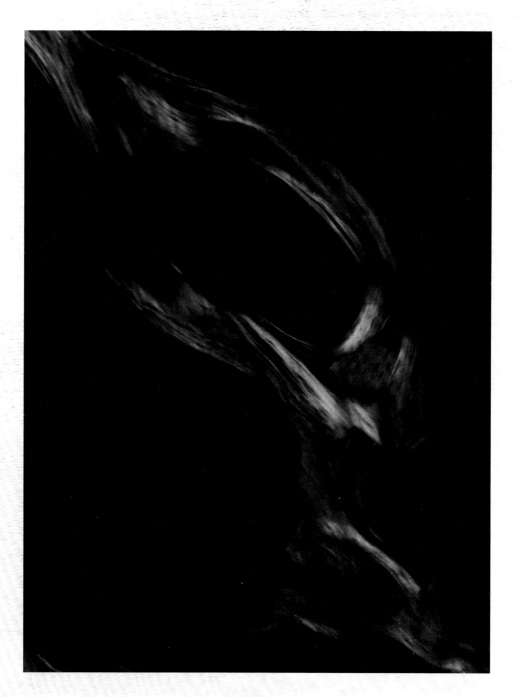

天书 No.112

未脱钙骨组织磨片，X40，偏振光，2019

Heavenly script No.112

Trabecular bone, Ground section, X40, Polarized light, 2019

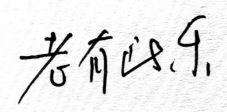

老有所乐

胡甲清，86 岁

The elderly have their joys.

Hu Jiaqing, 86

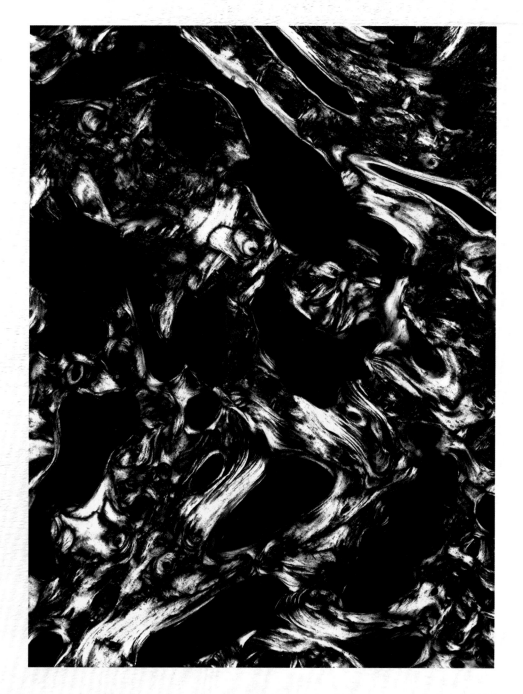

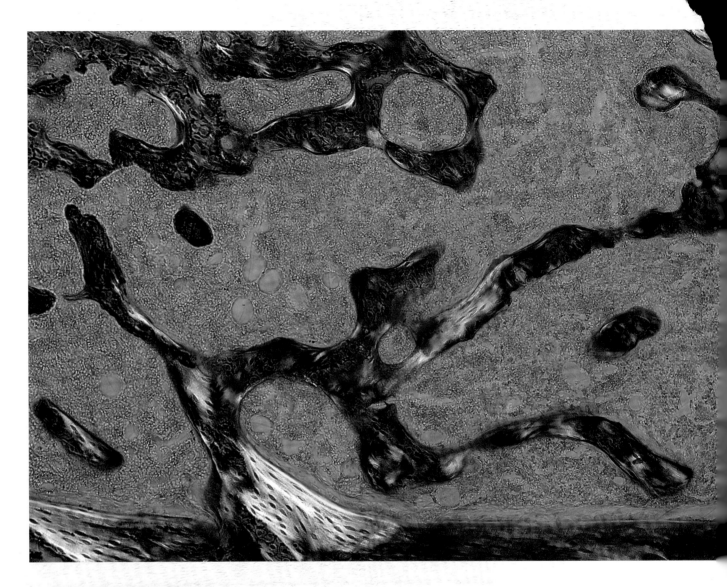

天书 No.106

未脱钙骨组织磨片，X40，明视野 + 偏振光，2019

Heavenly script No.106

Trabecular bone, Ground section, X40, Light field + polarized light, 2019

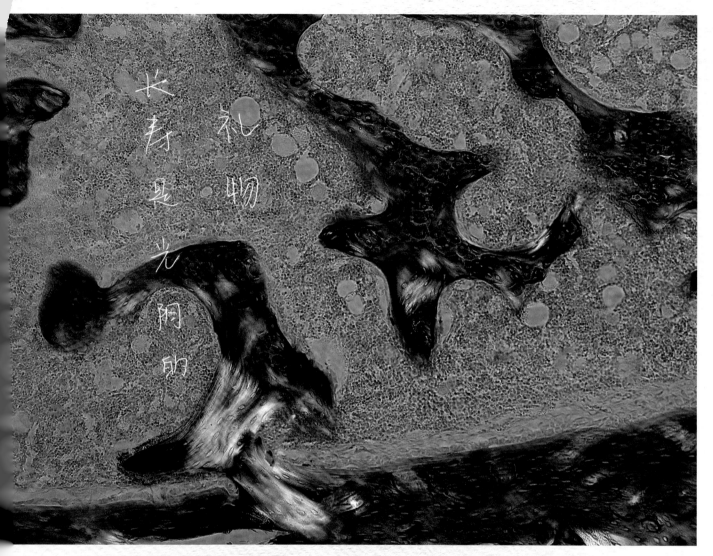

长寿是光阴的礼物

周立春，87 岁

Longevity is the gift from time.

Zhou Lichun, 87

天书 No.52

未脱钙骨组织磨片，X200，偏振光，2013

Heavenly script No.52

Trabecular bone, Ground section, X200, Polarized light, 2013

繁华落尽方自在

王检非，88 岁

Vanity is vanity.

Wang Jianfei, 88

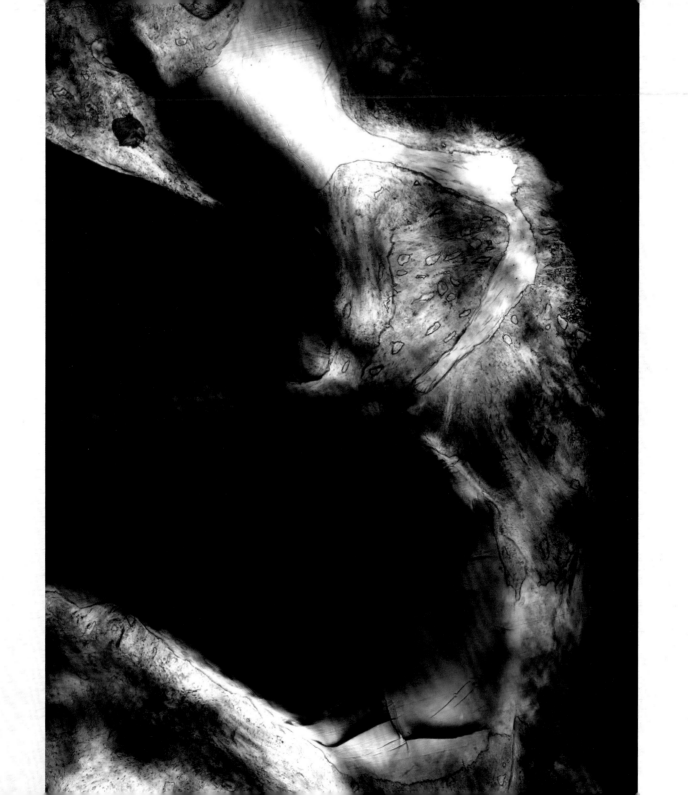

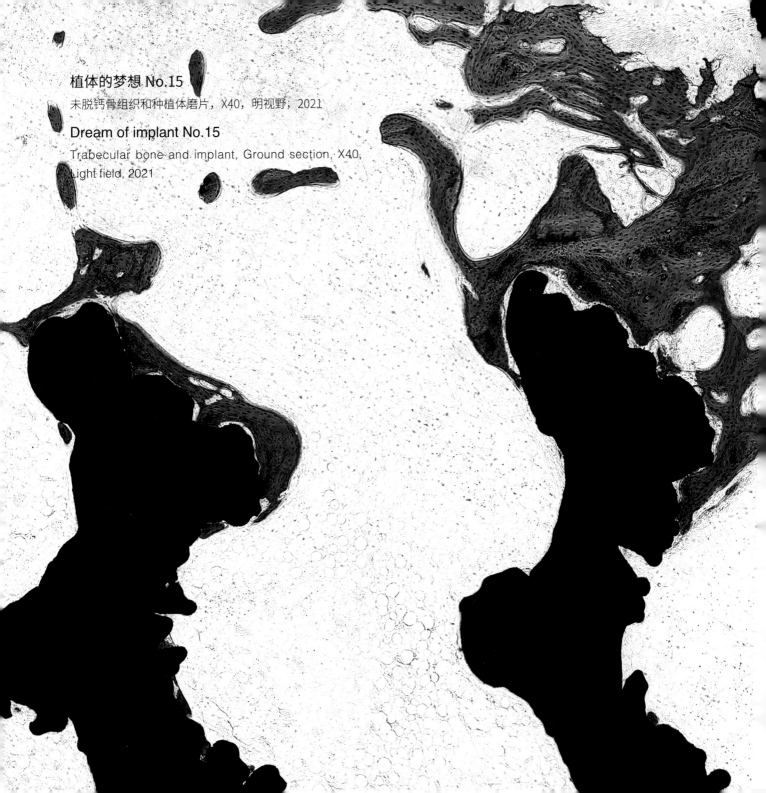

植体的梦想 No.15

未脱钙骨组织和种植体磨片，X40，明视野；2021

Dream of implant No.15

Trabecular bone and implant, Ground section, X40,
Light field, 2021

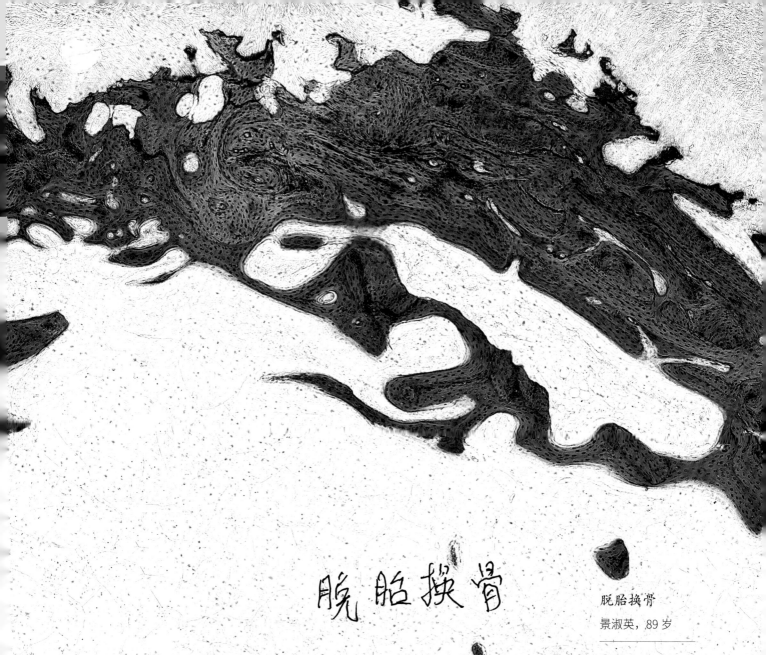

脱 胎 换 骨

脱胎换骨

景淑英，89 岁

Reborn to be a
new self

Jing Shuying, 89

凝固的时间 No.1

脱钙骨组织切片，X12.5，偏振光，2013

Frozen time No.1

Cortical bone, Tissue section, X12.5, Polarized light, 2013

高山长路，心中岁月。

吴世津，90 岁

Long road in the mountains, long time in the heart.

Wu Shijin, 90

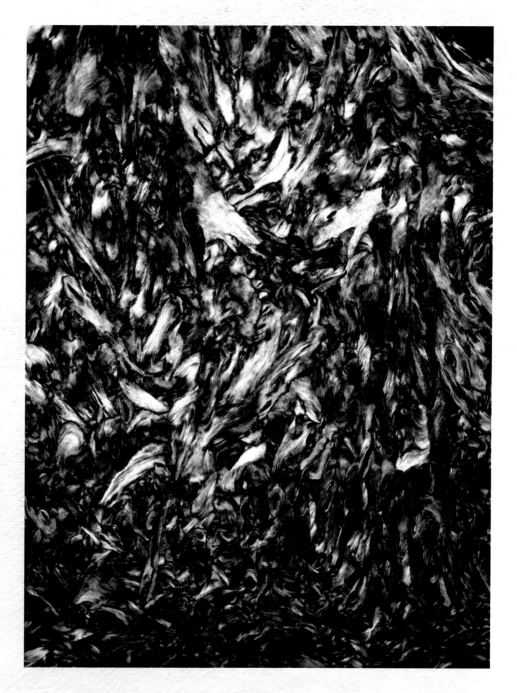

星球 No.2

脱钙骨组织切片，X200，偏振光，2013

Planet No.2

Cortical bone, Tissue section, X200, Polarized light, 2013

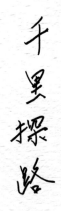

千里探路

宫心洁，91 岁

A thousand miles of exploration

Gong Xinjie, 91

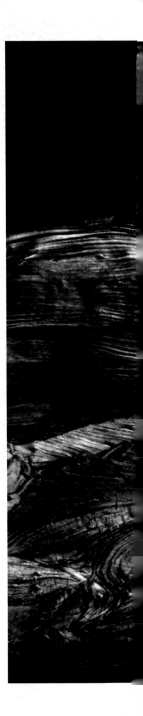

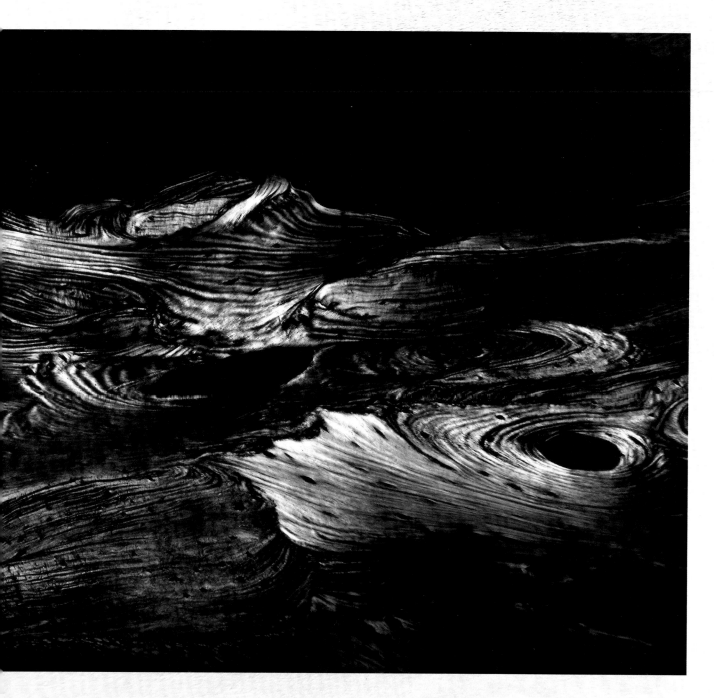

风骨 No.58

脱钙骨组织切片，X200，偏振光，2019

Backbone No.58

Trabecular bone, Tissue section, X200, Polarized light, 2019

轻舟已过万重山

轻舟已过万重山

范娇英，92 岁

The swift boat has sailed past thousands of hills.

Fan Jiaoying, 92

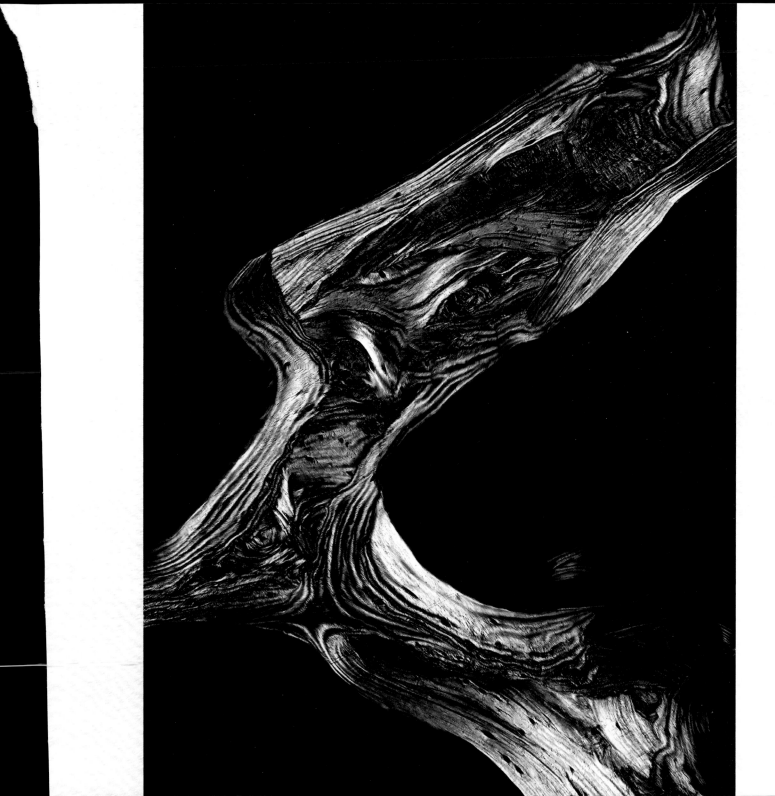

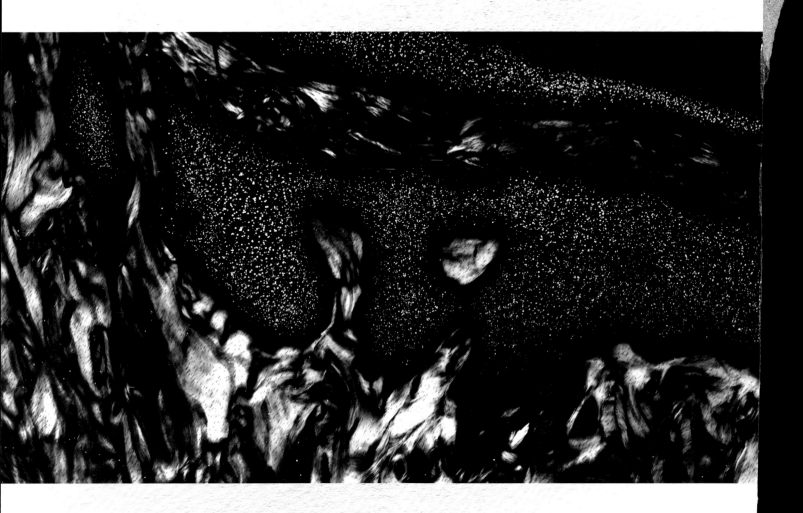

风骨 No.50

脱钙骨组织切片，X40，偏振光，2017

Backbone No.50

Trabecular bone, Tissue section, X40, Polarized light, 2017

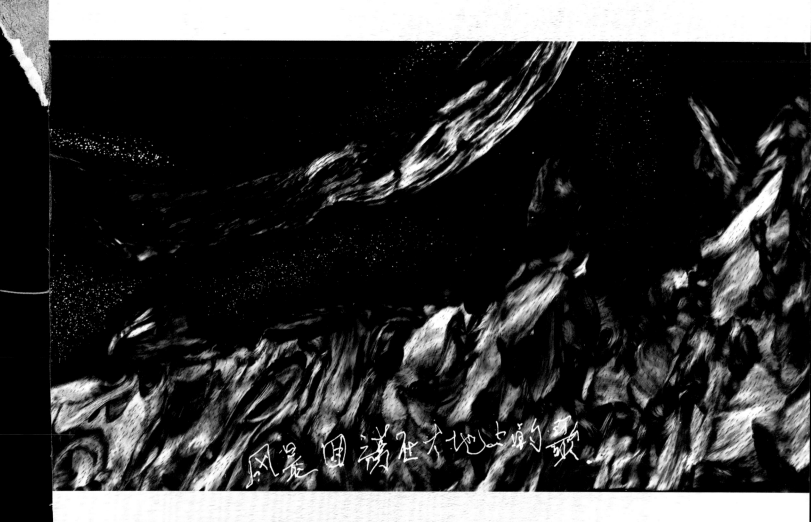

风是回荡在大地上的歌
栾玉英，93 岁

The wind is a song echoing across the land.
Luan Yuying, 93

风骨 No.36

脱钙骨组织切片，X100，明视野，2016

Backbone No.36

Trabecular bone, Tissue section, X100, Light field, 2016

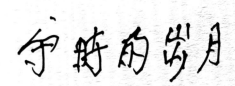

守时的岁月

吕春兴，94 岁

王雯，94 岁

Life is punctual.

Lv Chunxing, 94

Wang Wen, 94

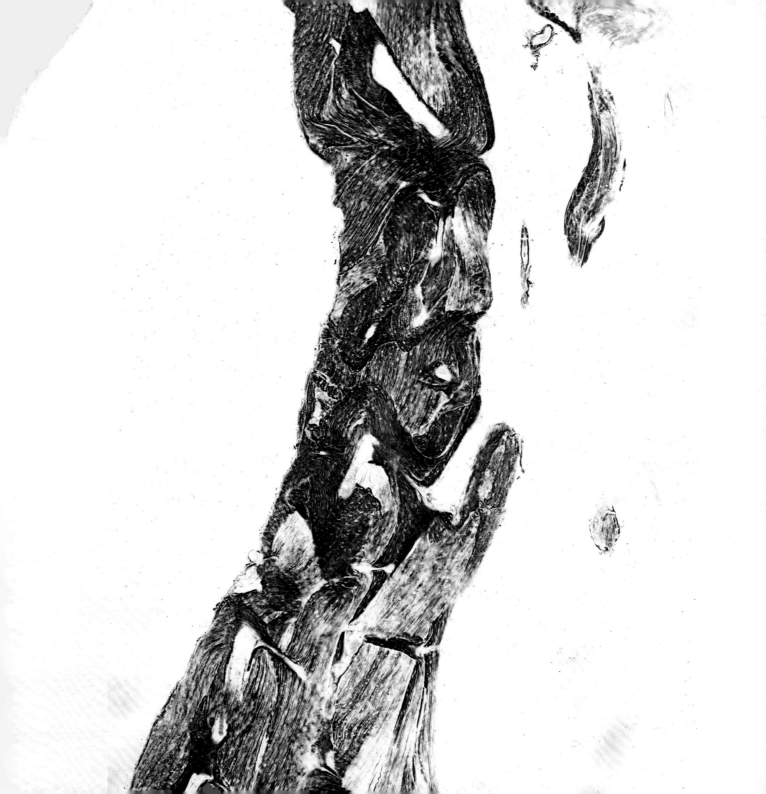

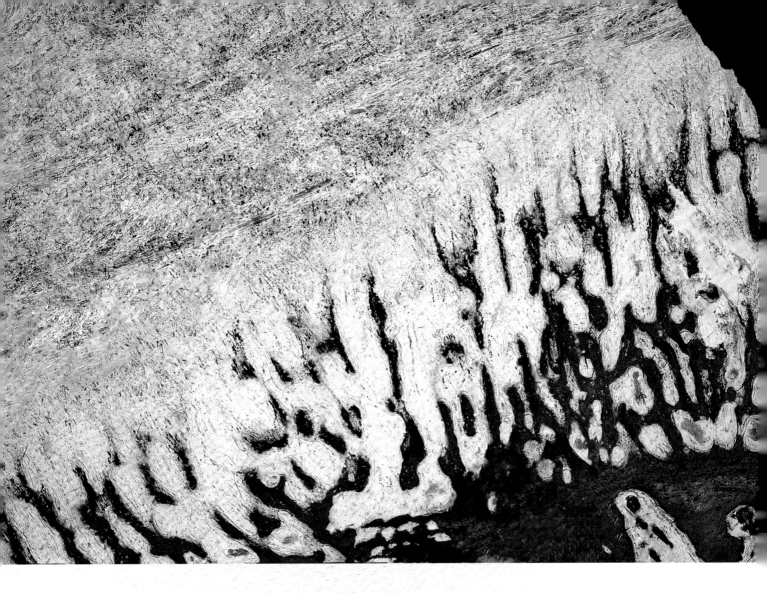

天书 No.186

未脱钙骨组织及周围的新生骨和软组织磨片，X40，明视野 + 偏振光，2021

Heavenly script No.186

Newly formed trabecular bone and surrounding soft tissues, Ground section, X40, Light field + polarized light, 2021

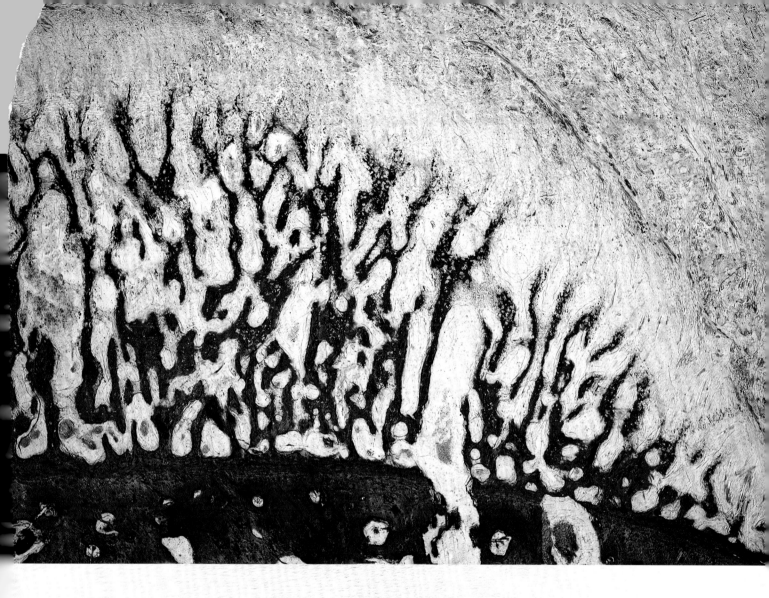

长寿时代

长寿时代

徐永德，95 岁

Times of longevity

Xu Yongde, 95

天书 No.179

未脱钙骨组织磨片，X40，明视野＋偏振光，2021

Heavenly script No.179

Trabecular bone, Ground section, X40, Light field + polarized light, 2021

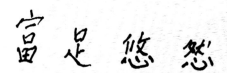

富足悠然

刑锡彬，96 岁
曹作郊，96 岁

Affluent and carefree

Xing Xibin, 96
Cao Zuojiao, 96

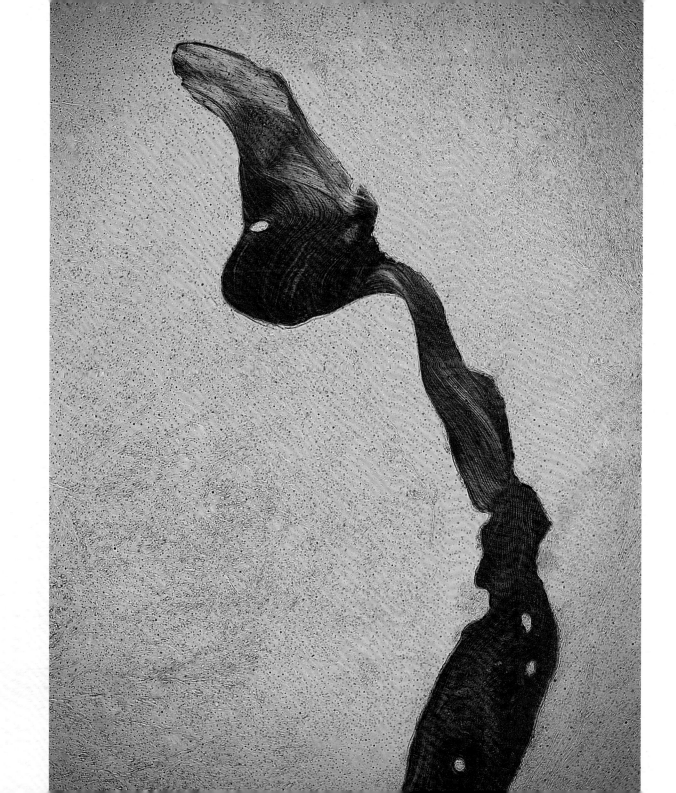

天书 No.180

未脱钙骨组织磨片，X100，偏振光，2021

Heavenly script No.180

Cortical bone, Ground section, X100, Polarized light, 2021

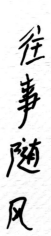

往事随风

郭静珍，97 岁

Gone with the wind

Guo Jingzhen, 97

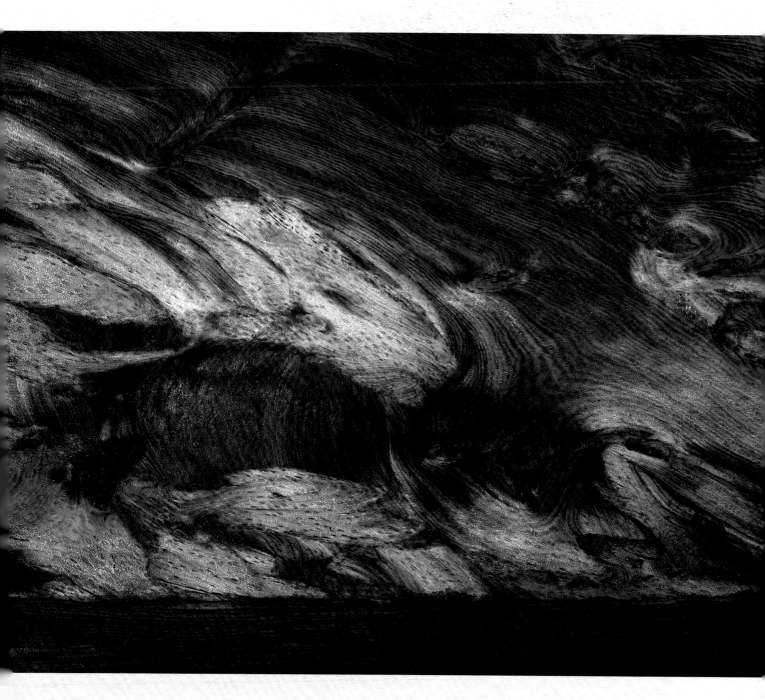

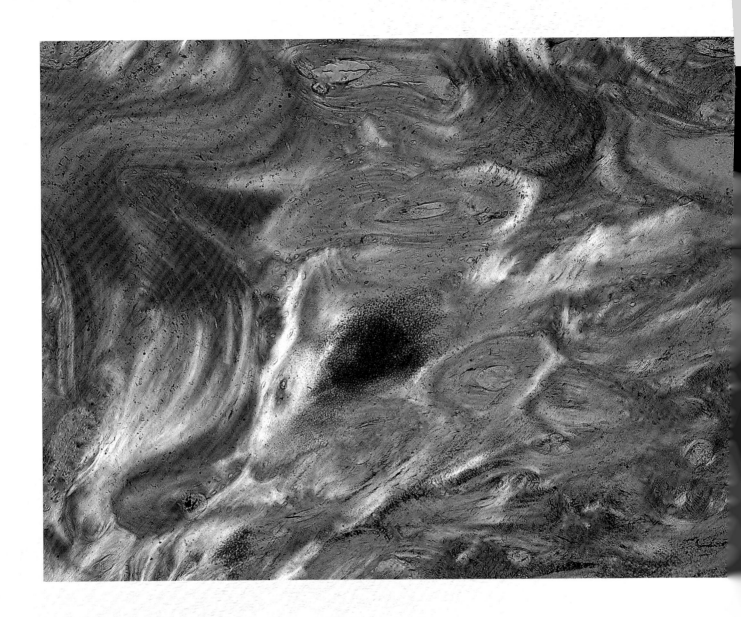

天书 No.176

未脱钙骨组织磨片，X100，偏振光，2021

Heavenly script No.176

Trabecular bone, Ground section, X100, Polarized light, 2021

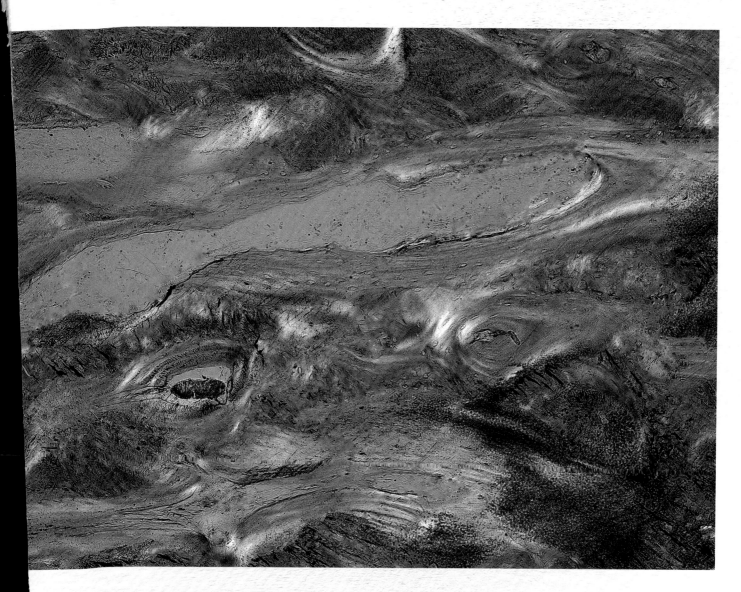

自己的光阴

葛殷氏，98 岁

One's own lifetime

Ge Yinshi, 98

自己的光阴故事

刘颐德，98 岁

One's own stories of life

Liu Yide, 98

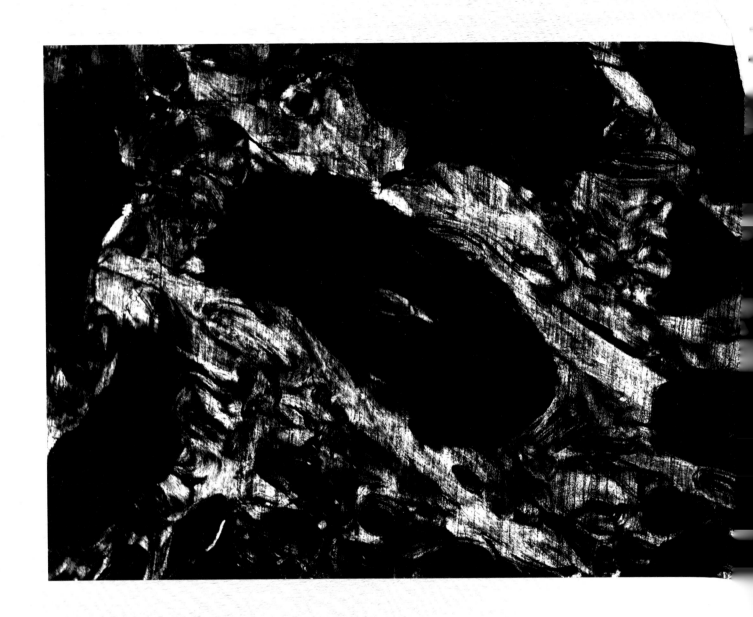

天书 No.133

未脱钙骨组织磨片，X100，偏振光，2020

Heavenly script No.133

Trabecular bone, Ground section, X100, Polarized light, 2020

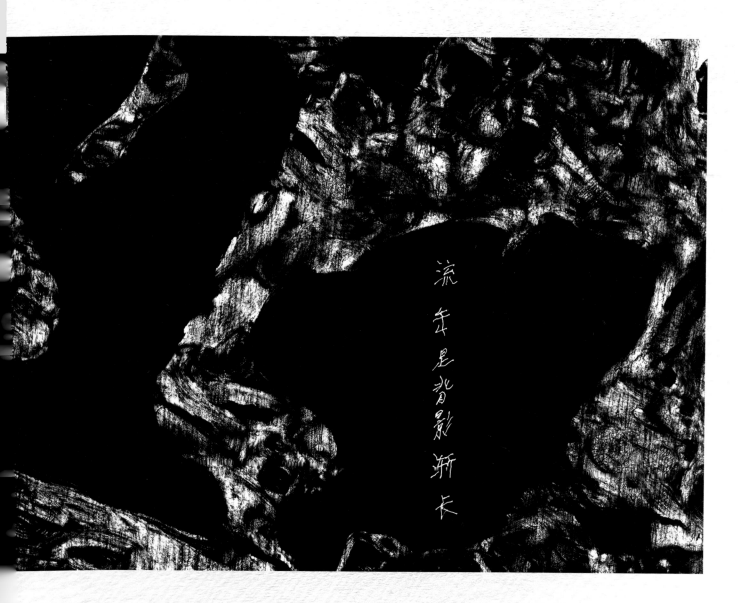

流年是背影渐长

张淑芳，99 岁

The shadow grows longer as years slip by.

Zhang Shufang, 99

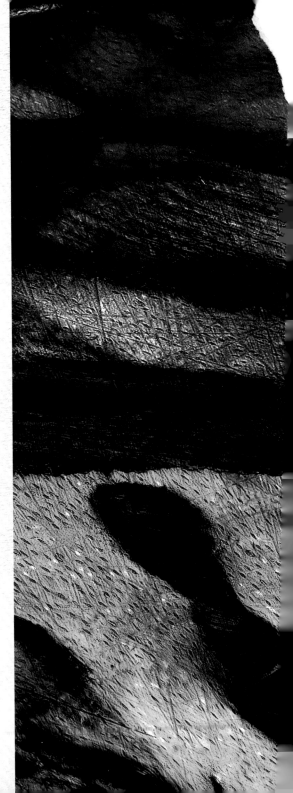

天书 No.149

未脱钙骨组织磨片，X100，偏振光，2020

Heavenly script No.149

Cortical bone, Ground section, X100, Polarized light, 2020

百岁不老

万国汉，102 岁

Still young at the age of one hundred

Wan Guohan, 102

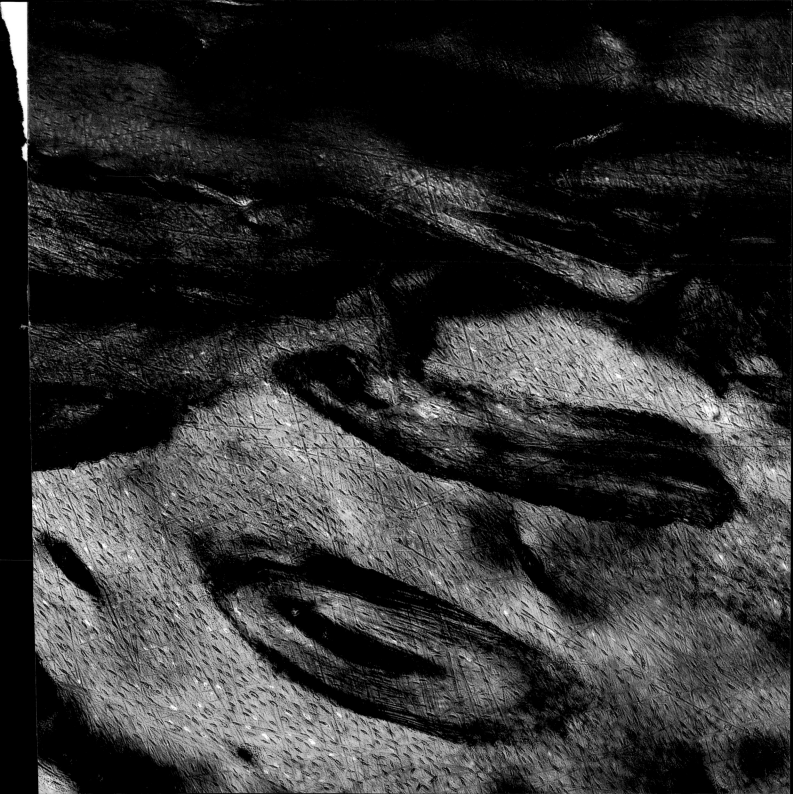

书写是生命的独白
——显微摄影艺术展观众留言节选

Handwriting is the monologue of life
— An excerpt of messages left by the audience at Li Tiejun's photomicrography exhibitions

生命如诗

李铁军显微摄影艺术展

北京大学医学人文周系列活动
北京，2013 年 11 月

Poetry in life

Li Tiejun's photomicrography exhibition

Peking University's Medical Humanities Week
Beijing, 2013-11

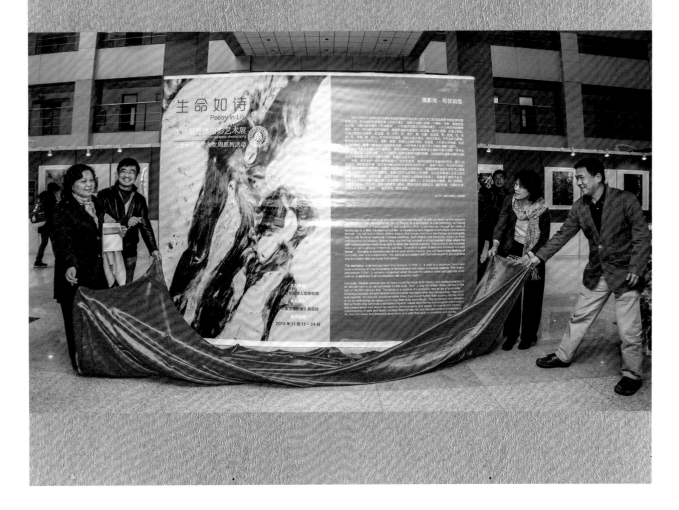

医学，不仅仅是关注病情的改善，它同样也关注人体的美。世界是美的，生活在这世界的生灵也是美的。一幅幅切片如达芬奇的画作一般美妙，热爱医学应从感受其美时开始。

— 医检-12
杜梦梦

显微镜下的时空是多元的，视野被无限放大，我们从微小的组织中看到了春夏秋冬，看到了生命如诗般绚丽。生命的河流将承恩，而医者将成为生之河流的护航者！

— 12级临床9班
刘雪娇

医学不仅关系到人类的生命安全问题，同时，也是发掘奇妙生命的开拓者。在浩浩宇宙中，医学由科技体现出的智慧是如此神奇。在宇宙之中，我们只是渺小人类。但生命能量体中，我们却也是团结的主力军，愿医学为人类创造奇迹，用科技带来光明。

— 11级护理4班
李冷

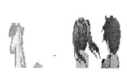

展览很有创意，给人耳目一新的感觉，从未见过这么美丽的切片。生活中不缺少美，缺少的只是发现美的眼睛。希望以后能有更多这样的展出。

科学往往是严谨的、严肃的，不容一丝犹疑与模糊的。这个展览为我们司空见惯的科学的组织切片赋予了美学的天性，变得抽象而朦胧，使人暇想万千。我们往往疲于分辨组织、分辨疾病，却未曾料到，科学也可以这么美。

11级 临床

生命不是细胞和神经构成，它也是一种艺术，在我们不经意之间，却展示于我们它的美丽，它等待我们去发现

11级 预防

以特别的方式展示生命之美。

13级 基础

看了这次画展，大师将人体的病变组织拍摄成了"春、夏、秋、冬"美丽的风景。不再是冷冰冰、令人害怕的病理切片。可见生活中处处存在美，令人厌恶的东西往往也会存在美丽的一面。

1311210025　高铧　基础医学院

平时显微镜下无情的切片被老师添加了许多美妙的含蕴义。照片很美，文字也很美，被老师发现美的眼睛感动。

1311210026　陈慕华　基础医学院.

于精深浩渺的微观世界吸取生命的瑰丽，虚实相生、动静相契。这些静态的、看不见的、写意的真与美，让人心生敬畏、尊重、感喟。这是医学从技术角度切割的艺术，是对生命的领悟与宏大的赞美。

—公教部2012级硕士研究生 陈燕婧
2013. 11. 15

观得抽空回到北区，就被大厅的展览所吸引，如果不是仔细去阅读介绍，我想这一幅幅的作品正如"春·夏·秋·冬"以及"风骨"～让我们看出了对大自然创造力的无限联想，"长河"、"燃烧的沙漠"它们好像出现在我们的眼前。然而当了解到这些作品都是四组以来色的时候，才发现这些被我们惊叹的美好原来就真实存在地存在于我们的身体里，原来我们每一个人都是大自然创造的艺术品，从宏观到微观，处处都是。感谢作者将这份最美的展示在我们眼前。在这一刻，自然·生命·人体是一个整体，而作者用一种艺术的形式展示出来。也在这一刻，医学也不仅仅是精益求精的科学，而是帮助我们去认识自然、认识生命、认识自身的一种方式。这种将科学与艺术结合的方式，让我在此刻很年轻，无享受这份宁静，这份温暖。

2009级临床八年制

2013.11.15.

　　参观了展览很是震撼，从没见有能这么美妙，进去在实验中本是的图片振影使用如此美的方式展现出来，太好了。多些这些展览吧。方也是一种从美的展示。

陈圆圆

2013.11.19

在浩瀚的宇宙中，我们的地球宛如沧海一粟。在无尽的历史长河中，人类个体的生命犹如同稍纵即逝的流星。然而生命是如此的曼妙，将这科学是这样的神奇。当我们用科学的眼光来观察生命，我们发现生命是的存在就是一个的奇迹；当我们从生命的视角来审视科学，我们发现科学也同样做为一门艺术在熠熠闪光。学科学，去探索未知的生命之道；欣赏艺术，欣赏光镜下我们自身的异彩纷呈。

—— 11医英·徐航

以往，我总固执地以为医学是严谨而理性的，医生是圣洁而超脱的，习惯了医学院相对沉闷而紧凑的学习环境，这样别出心裁的刺展无疑是给了我强大的心灵冲击。我也是喜爱艺术的小孩，却总在试图寻找一个关于音乐和医学事业的契合点，却总有一种业余爱好与专业相差甚远之感。看到口腔的老教授以如此美的形式完美的阐释了医学与艺术的结合，不由得有些心动，想想将自己的事业与爱好融为一体，大约是一件非常幸福的事！

—— 11口腔·张倩莉

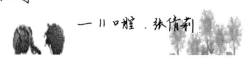

牙科的艺术

美国太平洋大学牙学院

旧金山，2016 年 8 月

The art of dentistry

University of the Pacific, Dugoni School of Dentistry

San Francisco, 2016-8

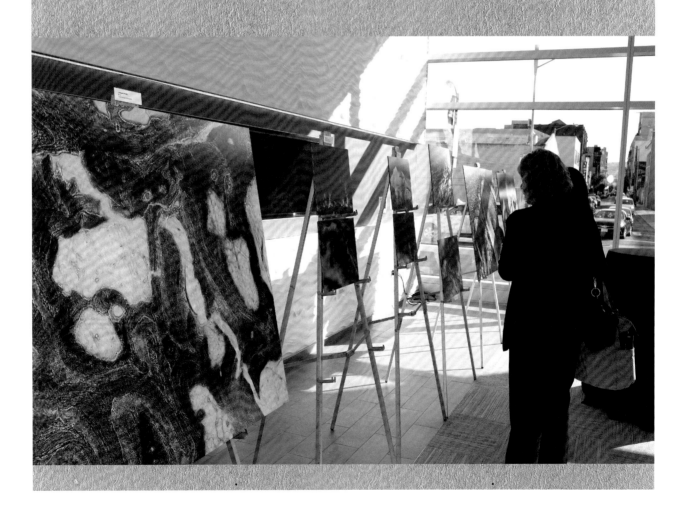

The ART of DENTISTRY

Photography by Dr. Tie Jun Li
August 12, 2016

The Art of Dentistry is a celebration and international showcase of clinical excellence. As a pathologist, Dr. Tie Jun Li is trained to assess the slides of blood vessels, teeth, muscle tissue, and bone tissue with an objective clinical eye. However, as a photographer, he could not help but appreciate the sheer beauty of nature under the microscope. This exhibit includes selected works from four themes in his photography: "Genesis," "Flourish," "Succession" and "Harmony." Together, they exemplify the true elegance in dentistry and narrate the cyclicality of life itself.

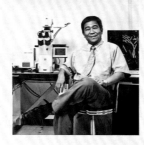

Hosted by the University of the Pacific, Dugoni School of Dentistry. A special thanks to the Peking Medical University, School of Stomatology and the Dugoni Global Relations Core.

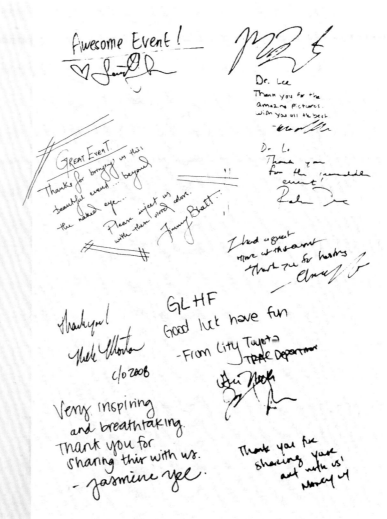

GREAT SHOW
QUITE INSPIRING!
— Karin

This was fantastic!
— Jen

Awesome Event!!
Great photographs, especially
loved the "starry sky"
Simply mind blowing.
— Nish
IDS 2017

Dear Artist
your art was so great! It
made me think of different concepts! Great
deb! keep on arting!
Always Rose G

Awesome pictures!
Congrats!
Rosmy Wesa

Congrats.
Mylie Mail

This was such a fantastic
Show, I enjoyed every bit
of it. PLEASE KEEP DOING what
you love. I am SERIOUSLY INSPIRED

THANK YOU!
— Revi Jin

Best!
Joann Marrow Cullen

Professor Li   Many Thanks for your
beautiful work & your
show in San Francisco
                Eugene LaBarn

Get content will
Sarcasm   Then Help D.S.9.

Silvan Wong 香望   Great job
Fabulous exhibit!   beautiful images
Congratulation!

热烈祝贺展览成功

中国驻旧金山总领馆

All the best!

Very nice to meet you
and your wife and son,
Beautiful work. Good luck to
you and your son's art career
            Jeff Joe

Congratulations!
    Deputy Consul General
    China.

Thank you for such
an amazing experience!
            - Kimi Loui
            c/o 2011

Good Job Rich!
        - Eric Ching

Congrats!
Susan + Erick
    Tonn

Welcome to
San Francisco &
Congratulations!

Thank you for such
an amazing experience!
            - Kimi Loui
            c/o 2011

Amazing
work
Dr. Farley   Sun Jia   Mary Liu &
                        James Wong

This is an amazing tribute to the beauty of nature. Art that we cannot ourselves [signature] Man Tin

I really admire your vision and pictures. They are showing multy of macro- and microscobbe beauty. Thank you for showing their beauty. Malabar [signature] Natasha Higherren

Best wishes
[signature] Donald Richau

All best wishes – great show!
Barry & Victoria Fong

[signature] U Ching [signature] M.D. Ret. Dr.

You are an inspiration as an educator, artist, and person. We look forward to more stunning work from you.

Congratulations!
Bill – Gloria Wong
[signature]

Congratulations!
[signature]

Thank you!
[signature]

please continue to make such awesome works for us to see!

THANK YOU FOR BRINGING YOUR LOVELY IMAGES TO SAN FRANCISCO. I AM BLESSED to BE ABLE TO SEE IT.
– JANE
[signature]

Amazing!?
Heesoo Oh

Well DONE!

Matthew Schuller

Amazing artwork. Thank you for being an inspiration to us all. Safe travels back to china, and we look forward to more of your work
- Laura Tsu

Best wishes!
P Christen

Thank you for the amazing artwork. We appreciate all that you do. We look forward to more gatherings like this.
-Sincerely GARY SIDHU
Max Saxton
Richard Hotchi

Awesome party!
John Cabos!

Go Dodgers!

Thanks for inviting us
- Molly's

Amazing
Echurs, I love the nature & histology metaphor. I'm a cell molecular biologist and I can relate a lot.
Best, Fernando R Curie

Thank you for the great job!
June Chang

Wow :)

S. Pidru.
刘长浩

Incredible artwork.
Thanks for sharing.
Gina S. Chann
阵晓
绍明
曾刚
一

Love the photos!
Joan Yokum

John C. Anygons

congratulations for your stunning show. we loved it! - Bill + June

Beautiful artwork!
SO IMPRESSIVO :)
横十健

Wonderful job!
Keep trying
Can't wait for next time
Val

Great Show!
J hm

Professor Li,
It was such a wonderful experience to enjoy your incredible artwork. Best wishes,
Prof Carpenter
(Bill) Carpenter

口腔新视界

寻境

武汉大学万林艺术博物馆

武汉，2019 年 11 月

The new vision of dentistry

Seeking new territory

Wanlin Art Museum of Wuhan University

Wuhan, 2019-11

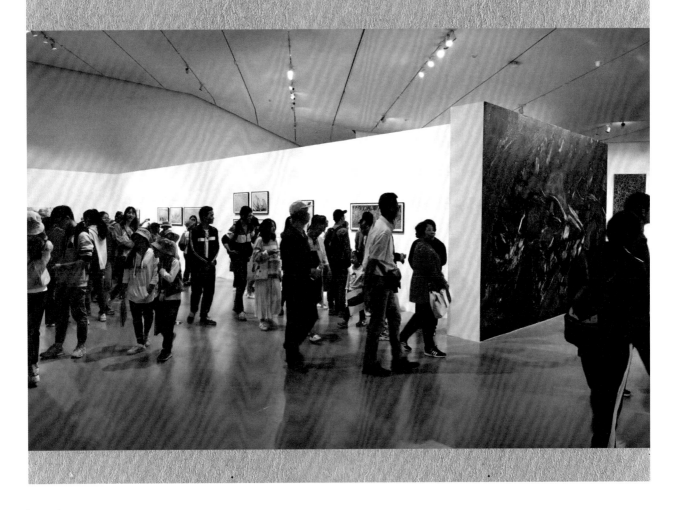

那些深深的感动

"我們淺淺地說"

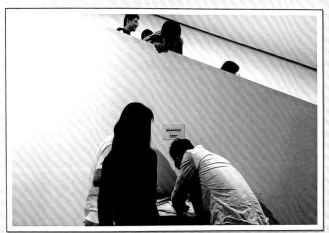

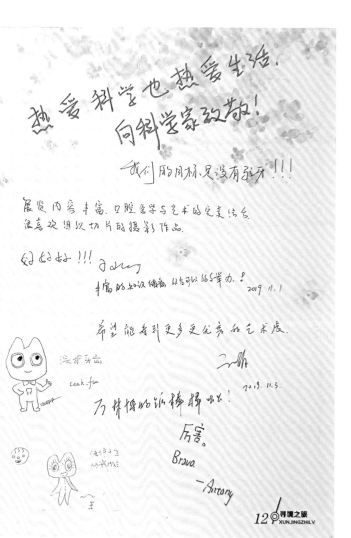

热爱科学也热爱生活.
向科学家致敬!

我们的月杯只没有张牙!!!

展览内容丰富.口腔医学与艺术的完美结合.
很喜欢组织切片的摄影作品.

继续加油!!!

丰富的知识储备,从何以6655学办!

2019.11.1

希望能看到更多更优秀的艺术展.

2019.11.3.

万林博物馆棒棒哒!

厉害.

Brava.
— Antony

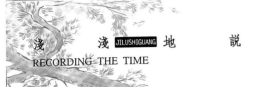

科学与美艺一脉相连、演绎一种别样的美才.
线条武大的邂逅才仰旦一场美丽的邂逅.
医科学更美!医科更棒!医武大更美.

19.11.5.

新西兰从湖南来到武汉.
觉得这个城市文化底蕴很深厚.
我爱武汉.

ⓔⓔ～

治疗的是牙齿
改变的是人生!

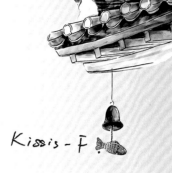

具有艺术特色.

爱了爱了

Kissis-F.

显微镜下也有一颗宇宙.

2019.11.08

希望自己在下学期开学成功转入口腔医学系
在自己热爱的事业上奋斗一生!

今年是自己一个人来的. 一个人看展览. 最近做了许多第一次的
事. 这个展览剃莉是改励自己的吧. 茶习期. 我还有我.
2019. 11.7

没想到我的嘴巴. 可以看见宇宙星辰. 治疗心录. 这个展览给我
更美好的看待世界的大途径. 只是一张口而已. 即拥有百物

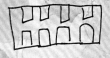

健康好牙. 健康知识教散 缘个.
Ryma.60.
2019. 11. 7.

打卡武汉大学

高科技
与
高素质

口腔医学 is very nice
从此喜上牙病的界...
武大外校来到一览

Hello!
口腔真奇妙!
我要好好爱护我的牙齿!
展览很不错!

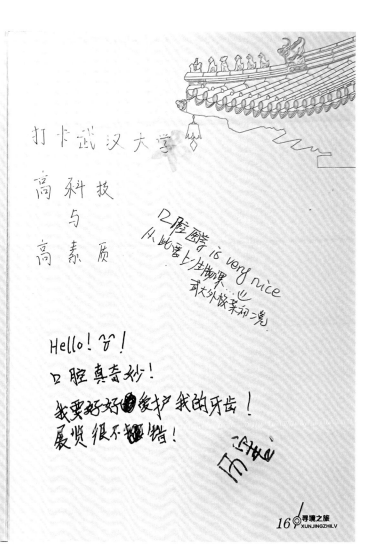

打卡武大

展览很棒！为艺术和科技都打开了
一扇新世界的大门！

when science meet art !

二层口腔新视界，科学艺术展非常有创意.
李铁军老师在摄影艺术方面
令人叹为观止.
也希望在2020年本科考试中.
我们能顺利考过.

钱军兄:

祝贺"寻境"艺术展圆满成功！
科学与艺术如完美结合.

　　　程鹏（82级口腔系校友）
　　美国·匹兹堡　11/13/2019

很棒！艺术性
专业性.科普性.
哲学性兼具！
时代的进步.
人民的幸福！♡

科学艺术❤
非常好 ☺
　　　—孟月涵 上小学

2019.10.9.

生物真奇妙!

教元乙
生きる意味とは何だ
教元乙

生命是一个非常奇妙的事物!!
——R.M.Y

切片很漂亮!

开阔了视野,
我第一次了解到生物岁的美妙!

牙口好也要疫

切片也能成为艺术!

我装到牙齿,特别是思想.

这个展也太精彩了吧!
微观艺术世界美得让人震撼!

祝我前程似锦

人从非洲来到武汉,
看到了这个艺术展,很震撼.

希望可以好好学习,天天向上,考上自己理想的院校.

牛! ——L.J.X

艺术馆去诸葛镇训了两次
可能更确是梦中偶核的力量吧.

——非洲的新生

关于作者

　　李铁军，1984 年毕业于武汉大学口腔医学院，1987 年获武汉大学口腔病理学硕士学位，1995 年获英国伯明翰大学牙学院博士学位，1995—1998 年赴日本鹿儿岛大学齿学部从事博士后研究。现任北京大学口腔医学院教授、博士生导师，兼任中华口腔医学会常务理事、口腔生物医学专业委员会主任委员、口腔病理学专业委员会副主任委员、口腔医学教育专委会副主任委员等职。李铁军教授业余爱好摄影，是中国摄影家协会会员，先后出版《生命之美：显微摄影写意集》、《显微镜下：生命的奥秘与遐想》（与彭志翔合著）、《寻境：生命之美显微摄影艺术》和《生命如诗如歌：显微镜下的人生四季》等有关显微摄影的艺术画册和人文专著。在国内外大学和艺术博物馆举办数次个人影展，其显微摄影作品在多种摄影专业期刊和媒体上发表。

　　黄慧萍，现任北京大学口腔医院正畸科护士长，副主任护师，本科学历。专业特长为正畸护理与口腔健康管理，先后发表学术论文 12 篇，参编护理专著 8 部。1992—1998 年随丈夫赴英国和日本学习、工作期间，在英国伯明翰 Chaplin 语言学校学习英语并获英语中级资格证书，在日本鹿儿岛 Akazika 学院学习日语并获外国人日语能力考试一级证书。

About the authors

Li Tiejun graduated from Wuhan University School of Stomatology in 1984 and subsequently obtained a master's degree in oral pathology in 1987. In 1995, he won his Ph.D. at the University of Birmingham (UK). He then worked as a postdoctoral fellow in Kagoshima University Dental School (Japan) during 1995-1998. He is currently a professor of Peking University School of Stomatology. Dr. Li Tiejun is also a photography amateur and a member of the China Photographers Association. He has published a number of art albums and books that combines medical photomicrography with artistic presentation, such as *The Beauty of Life*, *Under the Microscope* (co-authored with Peng Zhixiang), and *Seeking New Territory: Beauty of Life Photomicrography*. Several art exhibitions of his photomicrographs have been held at universities at home and abroad as well as in many art museums. His artworks have been widely distributed in a variety of professional photography journals and media in China.

Huang Huiping is currently the head nurse in the department of orthodontics, Peking University School of Stomatology. Her professional specialties include orthodontic patient care and oral health management. She has published 12 academic papers and contributed to the compilation of 8 books. From 1992 to 1998, she studied English at Birmingham Chaplin Language School in the UK, and later learned Japanese at Kagoshima Akazika College in Japan and obtained her foreign language certificates respectively.

李铁军已出版的显微摄影著作

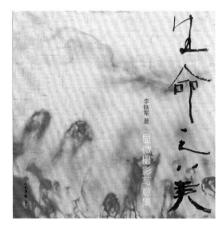

《生命之美：显微摄影写意集》，2014 年

The Beauty of Life, 2014

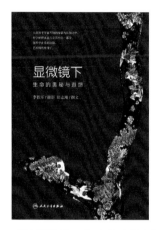

《显微镜下：生命的奥秘与遐想》，2020 年

Under the Microscope, 2020

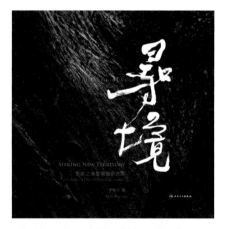

《寻境：生命之美显微摄影艺术》，2021 年

Seeking New Territory: Beauty of Life Photomicrography, 2021

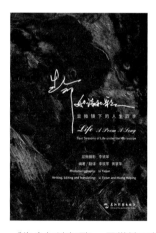

《生命如诗如歌：显微镜下的人生四季》，2022 年

Life, A Poem, A Song: Four Seasons of Life under the Microscope, 2022